THE RISKY BUSINESS OF ADOLESCENCE: HOW TO HELP TEENS STAY SAFE—PART II

HEARING

BEFORE THE

SELECT COMMITTEE ON CHILDREN, YOUTH, AND FAMILIES HOUSE OF REPRESENTATIVES

ONE HUNDRED SECOND CONGRESS

FIRST SESSION

HEARING HELD IN WASHINGTON, DC, JUNE 18, 1991

Printed for the use of the
Select Committee on Children, Youth, and Families

U.S. GOVERNMENT PRINTING OFFICE

47-042 WASHINGTON : 1992

For sale by the U.S. Government Printing Office
Superintendent of Documents, Mail Stop: SSOP, Washington, DC 20402-9328
ISBN 0-16-037310-7

SELECT COMMITTEE ON CHILDREN, YOUTH, AND FAMILIES

PATRICIA SCHROEDER, Colorado, *Chairwoman*

GEORGE MILLER, California
WILLIAM LEHMAN, Florida
MATTHEW F. McHUGH, New York
TED WEISS, New York
BERYL ANTHONY, Jr., Arkansas
BARBARA BOXER, California
SANDER M. LEVIN, Michigan
J. ROY ROWLAND, Georgia
GERRY SIKORSKI, Minnesota
ALAN WHEAT, Missouri
MATTHEW G. MARTINEZ, California
LANE EVANS, Illinois
RICHARD J. DURBIN, Illinois
DAVID E. SKAGGS, Colorado
BILL SARPALIUS, Texas
TIM JOHNSON, South Dakota
BARBARA-ROSE COLLINS, Michigan
JOAN KELLY HORN, Missouri
JIM BACCHUS, Florida
DOUGLAS "PETE" PETERSON, Florida
ROBERT E. "BUD" CRAMER, Jr., Alabama

FRANK R. WOLF, Virginia
J. DENNIS HASTERT, Illinois
CLYDE C. HOLLOWAY, Louisiana
CURT WELDON, Pennsylvania
LAMAR S. SMITH, Texas
JAMES T. WALSH, New York
RONALD K. MACHTLEY, Rhode Island
BOB McEWEN, Ohio
MICHAEL BILIRAKIS, Florida
SCOTT L. KLUG, Wisconsin
RICHARD JOHN SANTORUM, Pennsylvania
DAVE CAMP, Michigan
FRANK D. RIGGS, California
BILL BARRETT, Nebraska

Committee Staff

Karabelle Pizzigati, *Staff Director*
Jill Kagan, *Deputy Staff Director*
Danielle Madison, *Minority Staff Director*
Carol M. Statuto, *Minority Deputy Staff Director*

CONTENTS

THE RISKY BUSINESS OF ADOLESCENCE: HOW TO HELP TEENS STAY SAFE—PART II

TUESDAY, JUNE 18, 1991

House of Representatives,
Select Committee on Children, Youth, and Families,
Washington, DC.

The committee met, pursuant to call, at 10:00 a.m. in Room 311, Cannon House Office Building, Hon. Patricia Schroeder (chairwoman) presiding.

Members present: Representatives Schroeder, Rowland, Evans, Durbin, Collins, Peterson, Cramer, Wolf, Hastert, Walsh, Barrett.

Staff present: Karabelle Pizzigati, staff director; Jill Kagan, deputy staff director; Madlyn Morreale, research associate; May Kennedy, professional staff; Danielle Madison, minority staff director; Carol Statuto, minority deputy staff director; and Joan Godley, committee clerk.

Chairwoman Schroeder. Thank you very much. I want to call this second hearing in a series that we have been running on adolescence, the risky behavior, and how we can deal with all of this.

Yesterday was the first hearing in which we talked about the range of hazards, and I think one of the very interesting things was we found the correlation that was going on among a lot of this risky behavior.

The question we have today is how parents and other caring adults can reach these young people with information that is understandable, credible and usable. That is our real challenge today.

Today we are going to focus on ways teens and parents can communicate more effectively with each other, with their peers, with adults, and everyone else about reducing this risky behavior.

As you know, art can be a very, very powerful way of reaching young people, and we are very thrilled to have the "Secrets" cast with us this morning, who will be performing and starting this whole series.

[Prepared statement of Hon. Patricia Schroeder follows:]

Opening Statement of Hon. Patricia Schroeder, a Representative in Congress From the State of Colorado and Chairwoman, Select Committee on Children, Youth, and Families

Today we continue a series of hearings on a range of hazards typical of adolescence. It is a matter of real urgency that we learn about ways to help our young people make choices that enhance their wellness and healthy development rather than those that place their well-being and perhaps their very lives in jeopardy.

As we parents and other caring adults, must acknowledge the need to reach young people with information that is understandable, credible and usable. At yesterday's hearing we learned that several risky behaviors tend to come in a package. We have known for some time that facts alone are not enough to change adolescent behavior; we know now that information shouldn't be dished out in one-shot, fragmented, problem-specific doses.

We will continue to struggle with what and how we teach our children about these issues, with how to impart the social skills they will need to make use of the information, and with how to motivate them to protect themselves.

Today we will focus on ways for teens and parents to communicate more effectively with each other, with their peers and with other adults about reducing risky behavior.

Art can be a powerful means of reaching young people. I welcome the SECRETS cast who will be performing for us today, and look forward to the testimony of all the young people, parents and providers who will help us grapple with these critical issues.

THE RISKY BUSINESS OF ADOLESCENCE: HOW TO HELP TEENS STAY SAFE

FACT SHEET

DRUGS, PREGNANCY, HIV, AND OTHER STDs THREATEN HEALTH OF MILLIONS OF YOUTH

- Eight million junior and senior high school students (nearly 40% of this population) report weekly consumption of alcohol, including 5.4 million students who have "binged" with five or more drinks in a row, and 454,000 who report an average weekly consumption of 15 drinks. (U.S. Department of Health and Human Services [DHHS], 1991)

- In 1989, 91% of graduating high school seniors reported having consumed alcohol, 44% had used marijuana, 19% had used stimulants, 18% had used inhalants, 10% had used cocaine, and 9% reported having used hallucinogens. (National Institute of Drug Abuse, 1990)

- Approximately 1.1 million teenage girls become pregnant every year. In 1988, nearly 489,000 babies were born to girls under age 20 and the birth rate for girls ages 15-17 was at its highest level since 1977 with 33.8 births per 1,000 population. (DHHS, 1990; National Center for Health Statistics, 1990)

- Of AIDS cases reported in the U.S. by April 30, 1991, one in five was among young adults in their twenties. The average latency period between HIV infection and AIDS diagnosis is eight to ten years, therefore, many young adults probably were infected as adolescents. The total number of AIDS cases reported among persons ages 13-24 increased by 75% between 1989 and 1990. (Centers for Disease Control [CDC], 1991)

- Three million teens are infected with a sexually transmitted disease (STD) annually. Nearly two-thirds (63%) of all STD cases occur among persons under 25 years of age. Adolescents have higher rates of gonorrhea and chlamydia than any other age group. Left untreated, these diseases may lead to pelvic inflammatory disease which can cause infertility or fetal loss. (CDC, 1991; American Social Health Association, 1991)

SEXUAL ACTIVITY INCREASES AMONG TEENS; MANY ARE UNPROTECTED AGAINST PREGNANCY AND STDs

- An estimated 78% of adolescent girls and 86% of adolescent boys have engaged in sexual intercourse by age 20. Among girls ages 15-19, 53% were sexually active in 1988, compared with 47% in 1982. Much of this rise is associated with increased sexual activity among white and non-poor females. Among boys under age 19, the percent who were sexually active increased from 78% in 1979 to 88% in 1988. (DHHS, 1990; Darroch Forrest and Singh, 1990; Sonenstein, et al., 1989)

- The percent of U.S. teen girls practicing contraception rose between 1982 and 1988 from 24% to 32%. Nevertheless, in 1988, more than one-third (35%) of girls ages 15-19 reported no method of contraception at first intercourse and 82% of pregnancies among teenage girls were unintended, compared with 78% in 1982. Among never-married males living in metropolitan areas, 58% reported condom use at last intercourse in 1988. (Moser, 1990; Darroch Forrest and Singh, 1990; Sonenstein, et al., 1989)

- A study of 222 African-American teenage crack users found that 96% were sexually active, 62% had sold crack, 51% had combined crack use and sex, 41% reported a history of STDs, and 25% had exchanged sexual favors for drugs or money. While the average age of first intercourse was 12.8 years among the study population, the age at first condom use was 14.8 years. (Fullilove, et al., 1989)

COSTS OF DRUGS, STDs, PREGNANCY, AND HIV ARE STAGGERING

- Between 1985 and 1989, approximately 40,600 youth ages 15-24 died in alcohol-related motor vehicle accidents. (CDC, 1991)

- The aggregate annual costs of herpes, gonorrhea, chlamydia, and pelvic inflammatory disease are estimated to total $8.4 billion. (CDC, 1991)

- In 1988, families started by teen parents cost an estimated $19.83 billion in AFDC (Aid to Families with Dependent Children) payments, Medicaid, and food stamp outlays. If every birth to a teen mother had been delayed, an estimated $7.93 billion would have been saved. Federal funding for family planning services decreased by 39% between 1981 and 1991, adjusting for inflation. (Center for Population Options [CPO], 1990)

- The estimated health care expenditures for a typical AIDS patient from diagnosis to death range from $55,000 to $80,000. By 1992, the projected annual costs of AIDS are as high as $13 billion, not including treatment with expanded use of specific antiviral drugs, such as zidovudine (AZT) for asymptomatic HIV infected people. (Congressional Research Service, 1990; DHHS, 1990)

FORMIDABLE BARRIERS TO PREVENTING HIGH-RISK BEHAVIOR AMONG YOUTH REMAIN

- Approximately 4.6 million adolescents lack public or private health insurance, including nearly one-third of all poor adolescents. Of the estimated 21.7 million adolescents who are covered by private health insurance, one-third are not covered for maternity-related services by their parents' insurance. (Office of Technology Assessment, 1991)

- Fewer than half (47%) of sexually active teens surveyed reported having talked with their parents about sex and birth control. Nearly six in ten (58%) of sexually active teens who have discussed both of these issues with their parents report consistent use of birth control, compared with 16% of sexually active teens who have talked with their parents about sex but not contraception. (CPO, 1990)

- A 1989 survey of over 4,000 public school teachers who provide sex education found that while 75% believed that a wide range of topics related to the prevention of pregnancy and infection should be taught before the end of the seventh grade, only 35% reported that sex education was provided in grades seven and eight. Virtually all teachers (97%) felt that sex education classes should include information about how students can obtain birth control, but only 48% were in schools where this was done. (Darroch Forrest and Silverman, 1989)

- During the 1988-89 school year, two-thirds of school districts nationwide required that HIV education be provided at some time for students in grades 7-12. Only 15% of school districts provided HIV education in grades 11-12, although rates of sexual activity are known to increase markedly during this period. One-fifth of HIV teachers reported having received no specialized training in the subject. (Government Accounting Office, 1990)

COMPREHENSIVE, INTEGRATED SKILL-BASED PREVENTION PROGRAMS SHOW RESULTS

- A recent analysis of 100 programs that were successful in reducing high-risk behaviors among youth found several common strategies: Intense one-on-one individual attention; social skills training; involvement of parents, peer educators, and schools; preparation for entering the labor force; and community-wide, multi-agency approaches to provide resources and reinforce messages. (Dryfoos, 1990)

- Participants in a comprehensive drug abuse prevention program for students in grades 6-7 were at least 50% less likely than students in a control group to use cigarettes, alcohol, or marijuana one year after the study. Parents of participating students were more likely to report reduced alcohol use and increased physical activity. The program supplemented peer pressure resistance skills training with parental involvement, community organization training, and promotion of local health policy change. (Pentz, et al., 1989)

- An integrated rural school and community-based family planning program in South Carolina targeting adolescents, parents, and teachers in graduate training yielded a 56% reduction in the estimated adolescent pregnancy rate. (Vincent, et al., 1989)

- Initial data from a study of 144 gay and bisexual youth indicated that 83% did not know that HIV can be transmitted during oral sex, 75% engaged in unprotected rectal intercourse and/or needle sharing, and 18% were chemically dependent. After participating for three months in a model prevention program which included an initial assessment, individual risk reduction counseling, peer education, and referral to psychosocial services, self-reported consistent condom use rose sharply (from 44% to 73%) and participants were significantly less likely to report oral sex and symptoms of dysfunctional substance abuse. (Remafedi, 1990)

June 17-18, 1991

***

Tips for Parents about How to Talk to Children About Sex

1. Parents are the primary sexuality educators of their children, and should begin to talk with them about this natural part of life when they are very young. Children want to discuss these issues with their

parents and want to hear their values. Do some thinking ahead so you know what you want to say about your feelings and attitudes. Your children look to you as a model, and your values provide them with valuable guidelines for making choices.[a]

2. The most important step you can take is to say the first words. Children do not always ask questions about sexuality, so you must begin.[a]

3. Try to answer your children's questions as they come up. It is never a good idea to tell children that they need to wait until they are older before you will answer their questions.[a]

4. Let your children know that they can always ask you any questions they may have.[a]

5. Teens need to know that sex will never hold a troubled relationship together. Fear of being alone is not a good reason to have sex.[b]

6. Let them know that decisions about sex should not be based on what others do, but on one's own feelings. Sex won't make anyone popular or feel better about himself or herself.[b]

7. Don't make the assumption that sex is your teen's major concern, or that sexual thoughts are only about intercourse. Tell your kids that thinking about sex is normal and that you know thinking about something is not the same as doing it.[b]

8. Adolescents crave privacy, but that doesn't mean they don't want you to be involved in their lives. Show that you are interested without demanding intimate details. Teens need to know you trust them.[b]

9. It's important for you to be honest. If you don't think your teenager is ready for a sexual relationship, say so and explain why. Teens need more than "just say no."[b]

10. Tell it like it is. Avoid fables, vague explanations, and untruths when talking about conception or birth.[c]

11. Give simple explanations. Use appropriate names for parts and functions of the body. Children need a language to use when talking about their feelings, ideas and concerns.[c]

12. Get to know your child's environment. Current jokes, the TV and news programs they're watching, their music -- these will provide unlimited opportunities to discuss sexuality issues.[c]

13. Separate the child from the behavior. If your child does something inappropriate, label the behavior inappropriate, not the child bad.[c]

14. Sexuality education doesn't mean teaching kids how to have sex -- sexuality is about body image, gender roles, feelings about oneself that carry into adult relationships, as well as reproduction.[c]

15. Build up your children's self-esteem. Recognize their talents, personalities and accomplishments, and avoid comparing them with others. Reassure your youngsters -- especially when they're going through puberty -- that they are normal. A strong sense of self-worth helps determine the kind of choices they will make, sexual choices as well as other important life choices. Children who feel good about themselves are less susceptible to peer pressure and better equipped to make responsible decisions.[d]

16. Don't be afraid of not being an expert. If you don't know the answer, admit it, and then find out. Or you and your child can find the answer together by sitting down with a book.[d]

17. Educate yourself about HIV/AIDS and other sexually transmitted diseases, and make sure your children have the information they need to protect themselves. For example, they should know that latex condoms with nonoxyl-9 spermicide are much more effective than other types of condoms.[a]

---

[a] How to Talk to Your Children About AIDS, (1989) Sex Information and Education Council of the U.S. (SIECUS), New York, University, New York, New York.

[b] Talking With Your Teenager About Sexual Responsibility, (1989) ETR Associates, Santa Cruz, California.

[c] A Guide for Parents and Kids, Talking Together About Sexuality, Governor's Council on Adolescent Pregnancy, Baltimore, Maryland.

[d] How To Talk To Your Child About Sexuality, (1990) Planned Parenthood, New York, New York.

Chairwoman SCHROEDER. Let me first yield to our distinguished colleague from Illinois and see if he has anything he would like to add at this time.

Mr. EVANS. No.

Chairwoman SCHROEDER. The gentleman from Illinois does not have an opening statement.

I understand that the young people would like to perform facing the audience. So what we will do if that is okay, we will go down and sit at that table, and we will watch. So come on up, and we will go down, and let's do it.

PRESENTATION OF "SECRETS" BY D'MONROE, APRIL JONES, KEITH KAPLIN, ANDY PANG, AND CHRISTY WINTERS; ACCOMPANIED BY JOSEPH A. GLOSSON, KAISER PERMANENTE, WASHINGTON, DC

HOTLINE. Hello. AIDS Information Hotline.

Can I help you?

CALLER. I've been dating this guy and I thought we were really getting close.

CALLER. Yeah, I have this girlfriend.

CALLER. But a friend of mine told me she saw him going into a, you know, a gay bar.

CALLER. But, you know, I also sometimes do stuff with guys.

CALLER. I'm sure he's not gay.

CALLER. It's not like I'm gay.

CALLER. But what if he is?

CALLER. But I want to be safe.

HOTLINE. Gay or straight, male or female, the virus doesn't care.

Any form of sexual intercourse without a condom is risky.

The only way to be absolutely safe is abstinence.

Avoiding intercourse and oral sex.

Hello, AIDS Information Hotline. Can I help you?

CALLER. My boyfriend, he always uses a condom, but the last time I think it had a hole in it. It was just a little hole.

HOTLINE. If a condom slips off, breaks or is torn, it can fail to protect against pregnancy or sexually transmitted disease such as syphilis, gonorrhea, and AIDS. So be sure to read the instructions on the package. I mean a condom is only as safe as the person using it.

Hello. AIDS Information Hotline. Can I help?

CALLER. Can't you get it from mosquitos? I bet you can, and they're just not telling us. Blood right? That's how you get it and that's what mosquitos eat.

HOTLINE. No, it's not transmitted by mosquitos.

CALLER. Don't tell me I can't get it that way, man. I know you can.

HOTLINE. If that were true, then a lot more people would have it because mosquitos don't discriminate.

CALLER. Well, this country's not safe any more. I'm going to go to a place that doesn't have AIDS or mosquitos.

HOTLINE. Hello. AIDS Information Hotline. Can I help you?

CALLER. Yeah, hi.

HOTLINE. Hi.

CALLER. All right. I'm really healthy. I mean I work out a lot, and I'm not sick or anything, but last summer I was in New York and I shared a needle with some guys. Now, it's not like it was drugs or anything. I mean it was just steroids, but I've heard about people getting AIDS through sharing needles.

HOTLINE. Well, AIDS is spread when the HIV virus is in the blood of one of those people using the needle.

CALLER. Oh, no, these guys were all really healthy. I mean it was a wrestling tournament, and since then I haven't shared needles at all. Well, once I shot coke with this guy at school, but he hasn't been sick a day in his life.

HOTLINE. A person can carry the virus without showing any symptoms. So there is a possibility you may have been infected. We recommend that anyone who has engaged in unsafe behavior, even if it's only been one time, be tested because early detection may slow down the effects of the virus. We also recommend that if you're sexually active, you take precautions to protect yourself and your partner.

YOUNG WOMAN. I've always been in a hurry. When I was two years old, I jumped into the deep end of the pool. They had to pull me out by my hair. When I was 12, I taught myself how to drive a car. When I was 16, I lied about my age and got a job as a cocktail waitress, until one night when my dad came in for a drink. See, I've always been in a hurry. I thought I was smart. I thought I was ready. Same thing with my boyfriend and making love. I figured AIDS wouldn't matter. Why wait? Now I wish I had waited.

YOUNG MAN. I don't have it. Well, they say it's negative. They always do, but I keep getting tested about every three months. My—well, my friend, well, he gets tested, too. I guess we think if we keep getting tested it won't happen to us. My friends at school don't know. I mean I don't want to be treated different just because I'm gay, but it's definitely not easy keeping a secret like this.

ENSEMBLE. Secrets.
You have secrets.
We all do.
You're out there in your lives,
thinking stuff,
and doing stuff,
wanting to do stuff,
that you don't tell anybody.
You have secrets with each other,
from each other,
about each other.
You keep secrets from your parents,
from your teachers,
and friends.
You even keep secrets from yourself.
There are some things
you aren't ever going to let yourself know,
and you already know
what those secrets are.
Somewhere inside
You know them.

DENISE. I can't believe you're going to do this.

MONICA. Hey, this is how my mom and dad did it. They went on dates.

DENISE. You want to marry this guy?

MONICA. How do I know what I want? But I'm sick of meeting guys at parties. They have a few beers, and all they want to do is sleep with you. If Eddie likes me, he's going to have to get to know me on my terms.

DENISE. Oh, and then you'll go to bed with him.

MONICA. Sometimes you are so shallow.

DENISE. No, look. I'm serious. If you really like this guy, you should be prepared.

MONICA. Prepared? Prepared for what?

DENISE. Being naive is not a very good form of birth control. Look. I use two kinds. You should always have a back-up.

MONICA. Condoms. I heard———

DENISE. A rubber? Are you kidding?

MONICA. Denise, I'm not kidding. You should know this. A condom is the only way to protect yourself from, you know, diseases.

DENISE. Yeah, but———

MONICA. That's not all. The condom has to be latex and lubricated with non-oxynol-9. Well, anyway, I like Eddie. I'm going out with him, but that's it. There are other ways to get to know somebody without having sex with them.

DENISE. You might as well have sex with him. Everybody's going to think you are anyway.

MONICA. Who cares what everybody things? Denise, he has a choice, and I have a choice, and I'm choosing not to sleep with him.

HOTLINE. Hello. AIDS Information Hotline. Can I help you?

EDDIE. I've tested positive for the AIDS antibodies, and I don't know what to do.

HOTLINE. Well, there's a lot you can do to stay healthy. If you would like, you can come in and we can talk. It would also be a good idea to inform any sexual partners and, if you've shared a needle in the past, those people should be notified as well.

EDDIE. Just one time in New York. Well, there was this guy at school, but it was only once. You don't think I gave it to him, do you?

HOTLINE. Hello. AIDS Information Hotline. Can I help you?

CALLER. I shot up with this kid at school, and I thought he was clean, but he just tested positive.

CALLER. Yes, I'm sure it's nothing serious, but I've occasionally shared needles in the past. They seemed really nice. Now I've got these white spots inside my mouth. I think it might be thrush, but it won't go away.

CALLER. Is there some way to get it that we haven't been hearing about? I donated blood and it was rejected. They told me that I'm carrying the AIDS antibodies. What am I going to tell my wife?

CALLER. I always wanted a family of my own. When I met Duane, I knew it was right. And when I got pregnant on my honeymoon, I knew it was right. But when my baby was born, something was wrong. She—my baby has AIDS. She got it from me. I felt healthy and I gave no sign I was infected. Maybe I got it from the older man I dated in high school. Who knows? They say my baby won't live very long, but I can't think about that. I spend all my time with her. Even when she's sleeping, I hold her and hold her. She likes that. She also likes the stuffed rabbit my mom gave her, the song on the music box, and the sound of her daddy's voice.

HOTLINE. I wish we could tell you that these stories are fiction, that none of this ever happened, but we can't.

I wish we could tell you what became of the people that these stories are based on. We don't know.

What we do know is that stories like these are being told.

Or kept secret.

Throughout the country, in fact, all over the world.

AIDS is very hard to get.

You have to do something very specific to get it, either share a contaminated needle,

or have unprotected sex.

The point is that once you have AIDS.

you can't get rid of it.

There is no cure.

[Applause.]

AIDS is everybody's concern, but this play focused on teenagers.

Because at least one out of every five new cases of AIDS is someone between the ages of 20 and 29.

And most people carry the virus for years before they get sick.

That means that these new cases are people who are probably infected around the age of 16.

Which is why Kaiser Permanente presents the full production of "Secrets" at no charge to high school assemblies on a daily basis.

The most important part of the play comes at this time when we usually give the students a chance to ask any questions that they would like. We would like to give you that same opportunity, but first we would like to introduce ourselves.

Mr. KAPLIN. I am Keith.

Mr. D'MONROE. I am D'Monroe.

Ms. JONES. My name is April.

Mr. PANG. I'm Andy.

Ms. WINTERS. I'm Christy.

PARTICIPANT. So we will switch places with you all.

[The statement of "Secrets" follows:]

(Actors move into place and sit.) (Music fade up from 0)
(Phone Rings)

HOTLINE

Hello, AIDS information hotline.

Can I help you?

CALLER

I've been dating this guy and I thought we were really getting close.

CALLER

Yeah, I have this girlfriend.

CALLER

But a friend of mine told me she saw him going into a, you know, a gay bar.

CALLER

But I also sometimes, you know, do stuff with guys.

CALLER

I'm sure he's not gay...

CALLER

It's not like I'm gay...

CALLER

But what if he is..

CALLER

But I want to be safe.

HOTLINE

Gay or straight, male or female, the virus doesn't care.

Any form of sexual intercourse without a condom is risky.

The only way to be absoultely safe is abstinence...

Avoiding intercourse and oral sex.

(Phone Rings)

HOTLINE

Hello, AIDS hotline. Can I help you?

CALLER

My boyfriend always uses a condom, but the last time I think it had a hole in it...Just a little hole.

HOTLINE

If a condom slips off, breaks, or is torn, it can fail to protect against pregnancy or sexually transmitted diseases such as syphilis, gonorrhea, and AIDS. It is important to use condoms properly. A condom is only as safe as the person using it.

(Phone rings)

HOTLINE

AIDS hotline. Can I help you?

CALLER

Can't you get it from mosquitos? I bet you can and they're just not telling us. Blood, right? That's how you get it and that's what mosquitos eat.

HOTLINE

No, it's not transmitted by mos...

CALLER

Don't tell me you can't get it that way. I know you can.

HOTLINE

If that were true, then a lot more people would have it because mosquitos don't discriminate...

CALLER

This country's not safe any more. I'm going someplace that doesn't have AIDS or mosquitos.

(Phone rings)

HOTLINE

Hello, AIDS information hotline. Can I help you?

EDDIE

Yeah, hi. I'm really healthy. I work out a lot and I'm not sick or anything. But, last summer I was in new York and I shared a needle with some guys. It wasn't drugs or anytrhing. It was just steroids. But I've heartd about people getting AIDS that way.

HOTLINE

AIDS is spread when the HIV virus is in the blood of one of the people sharing the needle.

EDDIE

Oh, these guys were all really healthy. It was a wrestling tournament.. Since then I haven't done it at all. Well, once with this kid at school, but he's not been sick a day in his life.

HOTLINE

A person can carry the virus without showing any symptoms, so there is a possibility you may have been infected. We recommend that anyone who has engaged in unsafe behavior, even if it was only once, be tested because early detection may slow down the effects of the virus. We also recommend that if you're sexually active, you take precautions to protect yourself and your partner.

(Music up then out.)

****

YOUNG WOMAN

I've always been in a hurry. When I was two years old, I jumped into the deep end of a swimming pool. When I was twelve, I taught myself to drive a car. When I was sixteen I lied about my age and got a job as a cocktail waitress, until one night when my dad came in for a drink. I've always been in a hurry. I thought I was smart, I thought I was ready. Same with my boyfriend and making love. I figured, "Do it now, why wait?" Now I wish I had waited.

YOUNG MAN

I don't have it. (Looks at result slip.) They say its negative. They always does, but I keep getting tested every three months. My, uh, friend, he gets tesated too. I guess we think if we get tested, it won't happen to us. My friends at school don't know; I don't want to be treated different just because I'm gay, but it's definitely not easy having a secret like this.

(Music on at level 3 or 4 when D' is in place)

ENSEMBLE

Secrets.
You have secrets.
We all do.
You're out there in your lives,
thinking stuff,
doing stuff,
wanting to do stuff,
that you don't tell anybody.
You have secrets with each other,
from each other,
about each other.
You keep secrets from your parents,
from your teachers,
and friends.
You even keep secrets from yourself.
There are some things
you aren't ever going to let yourself know,
and you already know,
what those secrets are.
Somewhere inside,
you know them.

****

DENISE
I can't believe you're doing this.

MONICA
Hey, this is how my mom and dad did it. They went on dates.

DENISE
You want to marry this guy?

MONICA
How do I know what I want? But I'm sick of meeting guys at parties, they've had a few beers, and all they want to do is sleep with you. If Eddie likes me, he's going to have to get to know me on my terms.

DENISE
And then you'll sleep with him?

MONICA
Sometimes you are so shallow.

DENISE
I'm serious. If you like this guy, you should be prepared.

MONICA
Prepared? Prepared for what?

DENISE
Being naive is not a very good form of birth control. I use two kinds. You should always have a backup.

MONICA
Uh, condoms. I heard...

DENISE
A rubber? Are you kidding?

MONICA
Denise, I'm not kidding! You should know this. A condom is the only way to protect yourself from, you know, diseases. (DENISE starts to interrupt.) Wait. There's something else. The condom must be latex AND lubricated with non-oxynol-9... Anyway, I like Eddie, I'm going out with him, but that's it. There are other ways to get to know somebody without having sex with them.

DENISE
You might as well have sex with him. Everybody's going to think you are anyway.

MONICA
Who care what everybody thinks? Denise, he has a choice and I have a choice, and I'm choosing not to sleep with him.

****

(Phone rings.)

HOTLINE

Hello, AIDS information hotline. Can I help you?

EDDIE

I've tested positive for the AIDS antibodies and I don't know what to do.

HOTLINE

There's a lot you can do to stay healthy. If you like, you can come in and we can talk. It would also be a good idea to inform and sexual partners and, if you've shared a needle in the past those people should be notified as well.

EDDIE

Just one time in New York. Well, there was a kid at school, it was only once.. You don't think I gave it to him do you?

(Phone rings.)

ALL

Hello, AIDS information hotline. Can I help you?

BOY

I shot up with this kid at school. I thought he was clean, but he just tested positive.

(Phone rings.)

LAWYER

Yes, I'm sure its nothing serious, but I've occasionally shared a needle. The kid seemed very nice. But I've got white spots inside my mouth and I think its thrush, and it won't go away.

(Phone Ring)

HUSBAND

Is there anyway to get it we haven't been hearing about? I donated blood and it was rejected. They said I'm carrying the AIDS antibodies. What am I going to tell my wife?

YOUNG GIRL

I always wanted a family of my own. When I met Duane, I knew it was right. When I got pregnant on my honeymoon, I knew it was right. But when my baby was born, something was wrong. She... My baby has AIDS. She got it from me. I felt healthy and I gave no sign that I was infected. Maybe I got it from the older man I dated in high school. Who knows? They say my baby won't live very long, but I can't think about that. I spend all my time with her. Even when she's sleeping, I hold her and hold her. She likes that. She also likes the stuffed rabbit my mom gave her, the song in the music box, and the sound of her daddy's voice.

****

ENSEMBLE

I wish we could tell you these stories were fiction. That none of this ever happened. We can't.

I wish we could tell you what became of the people these stories are based on. We don't know.

What we do know is that stories like these are being told

Or kept secret

Throughout the country, in fact, all over the world.

AIDS is very hard to get.

You have to do something very specific to get it.

Either share a contaminated needle,

or have unprotected sex.

The point is that once you've got AIDS

you can't get rid of it.

There is no cure.

(Move and bow)

AIDS is everybody's concern. This play focuses on teenagers...

Because one out of every five new cases of AIDS is someone between the ages of 20 and 29

And most people carry the virus for years before they get sick...

That means these new cases are people who probably became infected when they were about sixteen...

Which is why Kaiser Permanente presents the full production of SECRETS free-of-charge to high school assemblies on a daily basis.

The most important part of the assembly comes at this point. We introduce ourselves and then open the floor to any questions the students may ask. We would like to offer you the same opportunity.

Presentation to the
U.S. House of Representatives
Select Committee on Children, Youth and Families

Secrets

AIDS and Teenagers

by
Kaiser Permanente
Mid-Atlantic States Region

June 18, 1991

SECRETS OVERVIEW

SECRETS is a health educational theatre presentation for teenagers who are faced with increasing pressures related to HIV and AIDS. The **SECRETS** script was commissioned by Kaiser Permanente as a community service program. The **SECRETS** program is intended to increase student awareness of HIV and its transmission; reduce apprehension and prejudice arising from misinformation; and dispel myths and fears surrounding AIDS. The program also provides a forum for teenagers to participate in AIDS-related discussion.

SECRETS follows the story of Eddie and Monica, teenagers who must deal with their sexuality. Eddie has recently been involved in "risky behavior". Monica, and a chain of other people, figure in his journey from infection with HIV to living with the knowledge of a positive test result. The play shows teenagers how to develop decision-making skills for resisting peer pressure, discussing choices with friends, and communicating with parents.

Each 45 minute performance is followed by a 10-30 minute question-and-answer session which is led by the actors, who receive extensive HIV/AIDS information training prior to the tour. **SECRETS** is performed by troupes in six of the twelve Kaiser Permanente Regions: Northern California, Southern California, Oregon, Ohio, Colorado, and Mid-Atlantic States. Since February 1989 **SECRETS** has performed 1,119 times to 614,000 students in 737 locations. In the Mid-Atlantic Region alone, **SECRETS** has performed 177 times to 81,274 students and 5,593 teachers since February 1990.

MODEL FOR SECRETS PROGRAM DEVELOPMENT

When determining an effective model to create an AIDS education program for use in high schools, we naturally began with an analysis of the Professor Bodywise program used in elementary schools for general health education. The Professor Bodywise program is successful in a variety of ways. It creates a positive and enthusiastic environment for health education in schools, generates a powerful student response during presentation, and promotes a positive image for healthy behavior.

There are further advantages to choosing theatre as the means of communicating our messages.

1. Film and video have been used extensively to reach teens on a variety of issues. While these media are valuable, they pose several problems. Teens have become desensitized through television viewing to videos as an innovative form of communication. Videos are more easily made and distributed than theatre productions, but their actual use and effect are difficult to track. During a live theatre performance, we can see and feel our audience, both in terms of numbers and general effectiveness.

2. Live theatre also offers a unique opportunity to role model positive behavior using a peer-counselor model. Students see "real people" interact; people they come to trust. Teens can "see themselves" using the same behaviors demonstrated in the production, thus, vicariously rehearsing their own responses to similar situations.

In summary, theatre is a particularly effective educational tool because it demonstrates by example, establishes audience identification, and works on a variety of levels to stimulate discussion and create opportunities for other educational experiences.

Needs Assessment

Educational goals were defined by assessing the needs of our target group and environment -- ninth through twelfth graders in traditional and alternative school settings. Twenty-eight teachers and administrators from seven school districts participated in the initial written surveys and focus groups. Results of the needs assessment include these findings:

- 100% of respondents agreed or strongly agreed that AIDS education was needed in their schools
- 78% felt the production should be less than 45 minutes long
- Topics they felt to be of importance for their students were as follows, with per cent of respondents in parentheses:
  - Fear of and prejudice against AIDS patients (100%)
  - Transmission of HIV (93%)
  - Reducing the risk of contracting AIDS (89%)
  - Safe sexual activities including abstinence (85%)
  - Medical explanation of AIDS (82%)
  - Drug abuse (78%)
  - Self esteem (64%)

Through this analysis we concluded that schools and teachers were receptive to bringing AIDS education programs to their schools; however, there was some concern about dealing with the full ramifications of HIV infection in a school setting.

Program Criteria

The script was written and will continue to be evaluated on the following assumptions:

The program must

- be modern and up-to-date
- avoid euphemisms (i.e., "bodily fluids") that tend to obscure reality
- create real and believable "true stories"
- put the stories into the mental and emotional contexts of the students
- be short enough to fit in the school day, ideally 40 minutes

It will include

- the effect of peer pressure on decision making
- the ways AIDS is <u>not</u> transmitted
- acknowledging without encouraging sexual activity

Program Priorities

Program development priorities focused around five points:

1. Get the information to teens effectively
2. Personalize and individualize the threat of AIDS for teens. This <u>does</u> affect you.
3. Integrate self-esteem as an essential aspect in the ability to say no to risky behaviors
    - "just say no" is too simplistic for effective behavior change
    - Students need responsibility, not dictums
    - Provide concrete examples of how, when, and why to "say no"
4. Help teens understand the "chain effect" of AIDS transmission ("going to bed with every partner your partner has been with")
5. ASK more questions rather than provide all answers, encourage discussion, and provoke thinking for problem solving.

This strategy opens the way for the on-going educational process.

The script utilizes heterosexual and needle-sharing transmission for three reasons:

1. General attitudes and beliefs about AIDS include the sense that it only affects gay men. This assumption is clearly false for most teens.
2. Schools are more concerned about addressing heterosexuality as a primary focus in HIV transmission.
3. The sexually active gay teen needs a very different educational model than the bisexually experimental or heterosexual teen; we do not have the resources to address all of these adequately.

Development Advisory Committee

The program was developed by an Advisory Committee in the Kaiser Permanente Northern California Region. The committee intended to create a balance among educational experts, medical experts, experts on adolescents, community standards, and teen perceptions.

Sabrina Klein, Ph.D., Chair, Kaiser Permanenente Northern California
Specialist in educational theatre and school-based community service
Patricia Loughrey, Playwright, Specialist in teen issues, dialogue and situations
Charles J. Wibbelsman, M.D., Director of Teen Medicine, Kaiser Foundation Hospital
San Francisco; co-author : Teen Age Body Book
Wendy Cuneo, Ph.D., Consultant to Kaiser Permanente Central Office AIDS Task Force; AIDS education specialist
Michael Allerton, MPH, Kaiser Permanente Northern California AIDS Education Coordinator
Nancy Rubin, Berkeley Unified School District, Family Life Teacher
Katherine Kirkendall, R.N., Fremont Unified School District Truant Officer, Registered Nurse and Curriculum Coordinator for the District
Alissa Ralston, Marin AIDS Support Network Community Liaison and School Education Coordinator
Jennifer Eisenman, Teenager
Fred Jackson, Teenager

Funding

Funds for script development including research, needs assessment, advisory committee meetings, and commissioning of a professional playwright were provided by Kaiser Permanente's Northern California Community Service Program. Additional funds for start-up including original music, set designs, and purchasing of equipment were provided by Kaiser Permanente Central Office and the Sydney Garfield Fund. The Kaiser Family Foundation also provided a grant. Each Secrets Troupe is now funded by its own Kaiser Permanente Region.

THE PLAY ITSELF

SYNOPSIS

After an initial collage of informational telephone calls to an AIDS hotline, the play follows the story of Eddie, a teenager who "shared a needle a couple of times". His girlfriend, his father and a chain of people unknown to him all figure in his journey from HIV infection to living with the knowledge of a positive test result. The main characters role model positive decision-making skills, abstinence, resisting peer pressure, discussing condom use with a partner, and parent-teen communication.

LANGUAGE

Educational/Medical The language of the play is straight-forward when addressing medical issues around HIV transmission. It is explicit (expressed with clarity and precision) rather than graphic (described in vivid detail). For example, the script states that "vaginal, anal and oral intercourse are risky behaviors", but does not describe the actions involved in these behaviors. This does two things: 1) demands and invariably receives maturity from the audience, 2) acknowledges without encouraging sexual activity.

Characters The language of the teen characters in the play is generic in tone in order to avoid colloquialisms and speech patterns that could be condescending. The language is theatrically realistic rather that conversationally realistic so that focus remains on meaning rather than form.

SITUATIONS

To meet the goal of creating "true stories" and putting the stories into a teen context, the following situations were scripted:

The AIDS Hotline All the calls were checked with our local hotline for accuracy and presentation. The subjects were chosen as being most important for a teen audience. We deliberately intended to give a sense of the broad range of questions most AIDS hotline operators are trained to handle. Eddie calls Information/Directory

Assistance to get the phone number for two reasons: 1) to demonstrate how others can get that information, and 2) to differentiate his character from the other callers.

Modes of Transmission All modes of transmission in the play are based on true stories.

Testing These scenes are based on experiences in anonymous test sites.

THE PEER COUNSELING MODEL

The importance of peer counseling cannot be overstressed. The risk of "turning off" young people and thus losing their attention to the entire issue of AIDS prevention and awareness is always present. Since peer pressure and support are essential to the success of teen education, these concepts were built in the program in three ways:

1. The creation and portrayal of the characters themselves -- the main characters are teenagers who deal with much of the day to day reality of teen life.
2. The actor's appearance and presentation on stage -- the actors are carefully cast for youthful appearances and energy.
3. The questions and answer period led by the actors following every performance -- the full pay off for the peer counseling model comes after the performance. The students not only ask more probing questions of their "peers" than they are likely to ask of an "authority figure." but they appear to accept the truth and validity of the young actors' responses more easily.

Each of these elements is vital to the success of the peer counseling/peer role modeling foundation of the program.

Training in AIDS Education

The actors receive over 80 hours of intensive education in HIV/AIDS, transmission, care, and related issues from medical and educational experts. Training also includes watching videos on AIDS aimed at teens (both good and bad are useful), reading articles, brochures and books aimed at teens, and using the local AIDS hotline.

They also receive special training in handling large groups. There has never been a Question and Answer period that has gotten out of control. On occasion, there has been an uncomfortable pause, but it only takes <u>one</u> question to start.

In addition to the structured Q&A, the actors announce after each show that they will be available for those who have additional questions.

THE THEATRICAL PHILOSOPHY

The number of seemingly endless options open to the theatre are actually limited to just a few when education becomes its primary focus. Experimentation for the sake of artistic growth, an important element in professional theatre, is subordinate to the educational purpose of the program. Clarity and relevance take precedence over other options.

There are basically two approaches to reaching an audience as difficult to reach as teenagers (difficult because of their natural barriers to communication, especially with authority figures, and difficult because of their lack of sophistication in theatrical presentation). One approach is to take an emotional point of departure, trying to generate a subjective reaction from the audience this technique was a scenario intended to bring out anger, fear, pity or other strong emotional response. This approach is often called Stanislavskian after the actor and director who developed a method of "realistic" acting which focuses on releasing genuine emotions from both performers and audience.

The other approach is to take an informational, objective stance, trying to generate from the audience a thoughtful response based on a more analytical reaction to the material. This is often called a Brectian approach, after the director and playwright who believed in theatrical technique that cognitively affects both performers and audience members.

The **SECRETS** production has a deliberate push-pull effect, calling the audience to identify with individual characters and situations, then reflect on the consequences or impact of what they have just seen and felt. To this end, the theatrical "montages" follow emotional confessions or releases. The "chain" follows the date. The humorous "mosquito phone call" follows Eddie and Monica's embrace toward the end of the show. The moments of pure emotion still encourage analysis on the part of the audience.

In addition, audience participation is generated by breaking down the so-called "fourth wall" of realistic theatre presentation. The connection this generates between the actors and the students is an exciting and important part of the success of the program.

THE PRINCIPLE OF ENSEMBLE

The **SECRETS** script was created with an ensemble of five actors, three men, two women. This was done to reflect the statistical development of AIDS cases: while the majority of cases in the U.S. are currently white gay men, the percentage of cases in this group is decreasing. Among teenagers, the ratio of male to female cases is 7:1 (in the adult population the ratio is 13:1); in Africa, where the greatest number of AIDS cases are currently reported, the ratio of all male to female cases is almost exactly 1:1.

An ensemble, where a "group of complementary parts contribute to a single effect," was chosen as an artistic refection of the impact of the AIDS crisis on society. There are no lead actors, no good guys or bad guys, no one immune from confrontation with the epidemic on some level in today's world.

Secrets' Support For Schools

The process of bringing **SECRETS** to individual schools and school districts involves a joint effort on the part of both Educational Theatre Programs and the schools themselves. **SECRETS** has the advantage of being a self-contained program, and thus very simple for most schools to book. We provide our own sound system and stages, we require only enough light to be seen, and the play and follow-up materials are provided free of charge. We work closely with the schools to arrange the logistics of the performance, i.e., arrange special assembly schedules and performances dates that maximize the effectiveness of pre-existing AIDS curricula.

In many areas, **SECRETS** is the first AIDS education of any kind in the community. People have concerns about the content of the play, how to maximize effectiveness, and how to garner local support for AIDS education in the schools. Kaiser Permanente is able to support schools that decide to bring **SECRETS** to their students by performing at community premieres, involving local health workers, school administrators, and political leaders in reviewing the program, and participating in "information nights" for parents and teachers during which questions about **SECRETS** and AIDS can be asked and answered. We provide both a promotional video and a full length video on the show, and we attend meetings to provide information about the program.

One of the most satisfying successes of the program is the fact that the play is readily adaptable to special audience needs. We work closely with juvenile halls, drug rehabilitation centers, and continuation schools to determine how best to meet their population's needs. Sometimes this includes helping the school to set up an "AIDS education week," or going into classrooms after performances to speak more in-depth with students. In addition to the student brochures and teachers' guides which we supply, we have access to numerous community resources and are able to respond to requests for information about programs which address addiction, violence, peer pressure, and other problems which may concern teenagers.

The effect of **SECRETS** continues to be felt in schools months after the production itself. Many schools have instigated AIDS education programs because of the success of **SECRETS** with both students and teachers. We have heard numerous stories of students who have decided to be tested, received counselling, made major changes in the ways they communicate with their parents and peers, and changed the way they make choices because of **SECRETS**.

OTHER EDUCATIONAL THEATRE PROGRAMS

PROFESSOR BODYWISE'S TRAVELING MENAGERIE

The TRAVELING MENAGERIE presents eight health and safety messages to elementary school students in this 45 minute show. It promotes good nutrition, personal hygiene and an active life style; it addresses safety in the home and in automobiles; and presents the dangers of alcohol, tobacco, and drugs.

The play ends with the entire audience passing the Bodywise Star Test and earning a Bodywise Star. Each student then receives a Professor Bodywise Activity Book. Professor Bodywise has been performed 1,776 times to 567,603 students and 33,661 teachers in this region alone since February 1986. Nationwide, Professor Bodywise has been presented to 2,789,000 children in 6,194 schools.

NIGHTMARE ON PUBERTY STREET

In response to the suggestions from teachers and students the Northern California Region began piloting a new educational theatre program for middle school children in the Spring of 1991. **NIGHTMARE ON PUBERTY STREET** addresses such issues as body changes, family problems, and common anxieties.

KAISER PERMANENTE
Community Services

Kaiser Permanente's fundamental purpose is to offer cost-effective, quality, pre-paid medical care to the communities we serve. We believe that our health care delivery system is a community service, organized and sustained by individuals motivated by a social rather than economic vision; that we make a significant contribution to the health status of the community; and that our business practices are socially responsible and contribute substantially to reducing the ranks of the medically uninsured.

Strong support from loyal and satisfied Health Plan members and the community have enabled Kaiser Permanente to attain its pre-eminent position. And, we believe that the greatest contribution we can make to the communities we serve is to continue offering pre-paid group practice services as we have for nearly 50 years.

We also acknowledge that providing health services alone does not satisfy our inherent social vision or the expectations of Kaiser Permanente stakeholders. We have always been aware that earning the support and respect of the community required commitments that exceeded our principle mission to our members. Kaiser Permanente's success depends on the social, economic, and physical health of the communities we serve.

The community is our source of members, well-educated employees, vendors supplying high quality goods and services, physical space to function, and of legal and legislative policies that support our mode of operation. The community also provides the infrastructure to support the housing safety and transportation needs of members, employees, and vendors, as well as the quality of life that attracts and retains these individuals. To the extent Kaiser Permanente can help ensure a healthy community, we invest in the future success of the organization.

Therefore, it is in the best interest of the Program to become involved in efforts to improve the community's status -- investing material and human resources towards the amelioration of persistent and complex health and other social problems. While our concern should encompass the full range of issues being addressed by our communities, our distinctive competence as a health care provider suggests a focus on health-related projects, particularly in the area of preventive medicine and health education.

47-042 - 92 - 2

Appendix A
Background on Teens and AIDS

Teens are clearly and urgently at risk for AIDS. Between June 1989 and January 1991, the number of AIDS cases among 13-19 year-old Americans almost doubled from 389 cases to 646 cases. The number of U.S. AIDS cases occurring in adults 20-29 also increased significantly during the same time period from 20,545 to 31, 675, and now represents 20% of all reported cases. In view of the virus' long incubation period, many of these young people were probably infected while in high school.

The differences between teen and adult HIV transmission are outlined by Karen Hein, M.D. in an article published in The Journal of Pediatrics, January 1989:

> 1) more teenage cases are acquired by heterosexual transmission, 2) a higher percentage of teenaged patients are asymptomatic and will become symptomatic during adulthood, 3) a higher percentage of patients are black or Hispanic, 4) there is a special set of ethical and legal issues regarding testing and informing partners and parents of adolescents under the age of majority, 5) there are cognitive differences which affect the processing of information and differences in coping styles, and 6) there are special medical, economic, and social implications when teenaged mothers deliver HIV-infected babies.

There are three additional issues to be considered when focusing on teens: peer pressure is an enormous influence on behavior, teenagers are experiencing and experimenting with their sexuality, and there is a dearth of accessible and attractive education programs aimed specifically at teenagers.

Studies done by the Centers for Disease Control and the Johns Hopkins School of Public Health suggest that teens are either not being reached by AIDS education (now mandated in 29 states) or have not allowed their knowledge to affect their behavior. Ninety percent of the young people 12 to 25 who were studied knew how HIV is transmitted, and 86% were aware that condoms can reduce the risk of infection. Yet the majority had not changed their activities and admitted to such risky behavior as unprotected sex and drug use including shared needles.

The above factors were considered in defining our target group, recognizing needs, and planning for prevention education. For your reference here are some additional facts and sources on teens and AIDS:

- In the period from June 1989 to January 1991, the number of AIDS cases among 13-19 year-old Americans almost doubled – to 646 reported cases from 389. During that same time, the number of AIDS cases among 20-29 year-olds also increased drastically – to 31,675 cases from 20,545. (C.D.C. HIV/AIDS Surveillance Report July 1989 & February 1991.)
- These 31,675 AIDS cases among 20-29 year-olds represent 20% of all cases reported since the epidemic began. (Centers for Disease Control, February, 1991.) Considering that the lengthy incubation period of the virus may be eight years or more, it can be assumed that these people were likely infected while in high school. (Final Report, Work Group on Pediatric HIV Infection and Disease, U.S. Department of Health and Human Services, Nov. 1988.)
- As of January 1991, a total of 161,288 AIDS cases had been reported . Of these, 646 are adolescents aged 13-19. (Centers for Disease Control, February, 1991.)
- Adolescents experiment with sex and drugs more than any other age group and are more likely than adults to believe that they are invincible and immune to dangers from such activity. Repeated data from the American Medical Society and the American College of Obstetricians and Gynecologists reveals that during the past decade approximately one million unintended pregnancies occur each year among adolescent females.
- In a 1986 survey, 54% of adolescents said they have "no concern" about contracting the AIDS virus. (Pediatrics , 79;825, 1987)
- Several studies show that 90% of youths between the ages of 12-25 know the primary causes of AIDS transmission and 86% of them are aware that condoms can reduce the risk of AIDS, yet the majority of them had not changed their activity and still admitted to unprotected sexual and risky drug use behavior. (Medicine & Health, Nov. 21, 1988)
- Long-term behavior patterns for sexual and drug activity are formed primarily in early adolescence. A survey of 35,000 high school students across the U.S. revealed that: more than 50% of students 15-16 years of age were sexually active; 2.8 to 6.3% have used IV drugs at least once; and 15 to 43% reported having more than three sexual partners. (The Morbidity and Mortality Weekly Report, Dec. 2. 1988.)
- Sexually Transmitted Diseases (STDs) among adolescents are increasing at an alarming rate. In 1987, syphilis and penicillin-resistant gonorrhea spread faster than at anytime in the last 16 years. The U.S. Department of Health and Human Services reports that about 2.5 million teenagers (one of every seven teens aged 15-19) contract an STD each year. And, among teens aged 15-19, the reported cases of syphilis alone increased 8% from 1986 to 1987. (The Morbidity and Mortality Weekly Report, vol. 36 #54, Sept. 16, 1988.)

- Needle-sharing by IV drug users plays a central role in the spread of HIV among youth: it is a primary method of exposure to HIV for 15% of people with AIDS in the 13-19 year-old age range, and for 25% of people in the 20-24 year-old age range.
- The National Centers for Disease Control reports that more than 70% of teens in grades 9-12 in a recent survey believed--wrongly--that AIDS can be contracted through insect bites, by giving blood, or by using a public toilet.
- If current trends continue, in the next three to four years, AIDS will be one of the top five causes of death of youngsters between the ages of five and twenty-four. Medicine & Health, Jan. 1989.)
- Ninety-four percent of public school parents believe that AIDS education has a place in the classroom. (20th Annual Gallup Poll of Public Attitudes Toward Public Schools, 1988.)

Appendix B
Kaiser Permanente
SECRETS Information

Region/Coordinator	Performances to Date	
Northern California Region Carolyn King (415) 987-2223	Students: Schools: Performances:	211,268 303 407
Southern California Region Rick Burke (818) 405-3194	Students: Schools: Performances:	232,173 120 331
Northwest Region Mary Strebig (503) 721-6820	Students: Schools: Performances:	32,311 45 65
Colorado Region Maureen Hanrahan (303) 344-7260	Students: Schools: Performances:	26,569 54 81
Ohio Region Cassandra Wolfe (216) 749-8462	Students: Schools: Performances:	33,510 53 70
Mid-Atlantic States Region Joseph A. Glosson (202) 364-4660	Students: Schools: Performances:	59,854 124 153

Appendix C
Kaiser Permanente
National Perspective

Kaiser Permanente is a nonprofit prepaid group practice health plan providing medical care to more than 6.5 million members nationwide, or one out of every 38 people in the U.S.

Background
Founded in the 1930s by the well known industrialist, Henry J. Kaiser, and a physician, Sidney R. Garfield, M.D., Kaiser Permanente was established as an alternative to "fee-for-service" medical care for the wartime workers of Kaiser Industries. Today Kaiser Permanente is a national group model health maintenance organization (HMO). It is the largest and most experienced health care delivery system of its kind in the world.

Size and Growth
- The program opened for enrollment to the community in 1945, at which time membership was 26,000.
- The 12 regions are: Washington, D.C./Virginia/Maryland, Northern California, Southern California, Oregon/Washington, Hawaii, Colorado, Texas, Ohio, Connecticut/New York/Massachusetts, North Carolina, Georgia, and Kansas/Missouri.
- There are more than 8,600 physicians and 74,700 employees nationwide.
- There are more than 200 medical offices, and more than 7,000 licensed hospital beds, and over 200 medical office locations for outpatient services.
- More than 40,000 employers offer Kaiser Permanente.

Organizational Data
- A not-for-profit, federally qualified health maintenance organization.
- Management is structured as a partnership between the business managers of the Kaiser Foundation Health Plan and physicians of the Permanente Medical Groups.
- Medical care is provided by Kaiser Permanente physicians practicing in the Kaiser Permanente medical offices. Inpatient medical care is provided in some regions through Kaiser Permanente hospitals, and in others through selected community hospitals.

Contacts:	Daniel Danzig (415) 271-5953	Director, Media and Community Relations
	Linda Davis (415) 271-6430	Vice President, Public & Community Relations

Appendix D
Kaiser Permanente
Local Perspective

Kaiser Foundation Health Plan of the Mid-Atlantic States, part of the Kaiser Permanente Health Care Program, is a nonprofit prepaid group practice health plan serving residents of Maryland, Virginia, and the District of Columbia. The Capital Area Permanente Medical Group provides or arranges for the care of Kaiser Permanente members.

The Mid-Atlantic States Region was established on August 1, 1980, when Kaiser Permanente assumed responsibility for the Georgetown University Community Health Plan, a group practice prepayment plan formed in 1972 under the sponsorship of Georgetown University.

Kaiser Permanente membership in
the Washington/Baltimore metropolitan area: 280,000
Number of Physicians: 450

Medical Centers

Maryland
Gaithersburg
Kensington
Summit Mental Health Center
Camp Springs
Landover
Charles Plaza
Severna Park North
Towson
Woodlawn
Rosedale

District of Columbia
North Capitol

Northern Virginia
Fair Oaks
Merrifield Mental Health Center
Reston
Springfield
Woodbridge

Senior Vice President and Regional Manager, Kaiser Foundation Health Plan of the Mid-Atlantic States, Inc. — Alan J. Silverstone

President and Medical Director, Capital Area Permanente Medical Group, P.C. — Martin B. Bauman, M.D.

Contacts:

Stephanie Strass
Director, Public Affairs
(202) 364-3361

Jeannette Duerr
Senior Public Affairs Representative
(202) 364-3345

Chairwoman SCHROEDER. Wonderful. Thank you very much.

[Applause.]

Chairwoman SCHROEDER. Well, I want to congratulate all of you, and I think Kaiser Permanente is to be congratulated for having found a medium in which we can reach teenagers very directly.

There are seven troupes; is that correct? There are seven "Secrets" groups?

Mr. GLOSSON. There are a total of six, six troupes all over the country.

Chairwoman SCHROEDER. I thought it would be interesting to have you tell us a little bit about the reception that you get when you present this—from teens.

Mr. D'MONROE. Okay. Keith.

Mr. KAPLIN. Okay. Generally the audience, when it starts out, they might be a little bit noisy and do not really know what to expect from the presentation in school. But as we get started, I think we generally catch everyone's attention. By the end of the show, everyone is really paying attention, and we can tell how much people have listened basically by the question and answer period at the end of the show, by seeing what kinds of informed questions that we really get, that the show has sparked those questions.

Mr. PANG. And I think one thing that is kind of interesting about when we do the show, is when kids come up to you and they actually say that this is something great, is something that we really needed, that we needed to hear. I guess, people around our age give them the facts, give them the right information, just let them know exactly what is going on with the virus and give them the specific points on it.

Ms. JONES. Plus it is very entertaining. A lot of the kids tell us, "Oh, God, it was really good. We thought it was going to be another dry assembly," you know, because they are used to these really dry assemblies that they do not want to go to. So when we come, that is like Keith was saying sometimes they are a little noisy because they think it is going to be another——

Mr. KAPLAN. Lecture.

Ms. JONES. Yes. I mean you can hear it. They just really get quiet as soon as we start.

Chairwoman SCHROEDER. Well, you disseminate an incredible amount of information in a very effective form, and congratulations to Kaiser.

Does anyone have any questions? Yes, Congressman Peterson.

Mr. PETERSON. Obviously, you all cannot do this nationwide in your present form. Have you put a video out or something like that that can be put around to the rest of the schools?

It seems to me an important message, though you just cannot do it all in person in all of these rural schools and whatever. You need a greater outreach, it seems to me, in the overall.

Mr. GLOSSON. During the first 18 months of the program, as we said, it is in six Kaiser service regions. We, in fact, just obtained a grant to do a feasibility study to see about having a videotaped version of it done so that it is available in other parts of the country.

And one more thing. It is also available in a very specific basis, that groups can produce it. There have been six or eight different groups, University of Wyoming among them, that have produced this within a local community.

Mr. PETERSON. I represent a very rural district. I have got 25 counties along North Florida, and I have visited any number of those schools, and they just are not going to have the wherewithal to put something like that together.

I would suggest that you are not going to need a study to decide whether or not you need a video. You might need some money, but the study would be to me a foregone conclusion. But I would recommend that highly and certainly would invite in some way to get that out into my schools, into those rural schools. I think it is very, very important.

The problem out there is a shadowy figure. People do not realize that these rural areas have as much danger now with a lot of migrant society that we have. We are just as susceptible to this AIDS problem as the urban areas, in my view.

Chairwoman SCHROEDER. Does anyone else have a question of the cast while they are here?

[No response.]

Chairwoman SCHROEDER. Well, we really thank you, and I would like to underline what he said. I think the quicker you can make the videos and disseminate them, the better, because I really think that all of us could stand and give assemblies from here to kingdom come, and we would never be listened to as well as you are. It is a very, very effective way of communication.

Thank you so much, Kaiser Permanente, for sponsoring it and having the guts to sponsor it, and we want to thank, too, the very sterling cast. I thought you did just a phenomenal job.

So thank you very much.

Next we are going to call to the platform the Terrific PEERS Program, who we would like to come up and join us this morning. We have got Eleshia Ray, Kianga Stroud and Nkenge Toure. These are peer educators and a youth coordinator from the PEERS Program of Terrific, Inc., in Washington, DC.

And I want to say we are very, very happy to have you. It is wonderful to have young people talking to us this morning. After hearing all the problems yesterday that we are having with adolescents, we thought it would be interesting to see how adolescents are approaching all of these problems.

So let me turn the microphone over to you. Have you decided how you are going to proceed? All right. If you would introduce yourselves, the floor is yours.

STATEMENT OF ELESHIA RAY, KIANGA STROUD, AND NKENGE TOURE, PEER EDUCATORS AND YOUTH COORDINATOR, PEERS PROGRAM, TERRIFIC INC., WASHINGTON, DC

Ms. RAY. My name is Eleshia Ray, and I am in the Terrific PEERS Program.

Chairwoman SCHROEDER. Could you move the microphone a little closer to you? I am having a little trouble hearing up here. There you go.

Ms. RAY. Good morning to all of the members of the Select Committee on Children, Youth, and Families.

I would like to thank Congresswoman Patricia Schroeder for giving the PEERS Program an opportunity to be heard.

My name is Eleshia Ray. I am 15 years old, and this is the start of my second year with Terrific PEERS.

I know you are thinking, "What qualifies her to be an AIDS educator?" Well, we all receive between 40 to 45 hours of training, which we took over a period of five Saturdays. I learned all about HIV and AIDS transmission, prevention, testing, teen pregnancy, STD, and drug abuse. I learned about peer pressure, good decision-making skills, self-esteem and leadership.

The program also taught me how to prepare presentations and do public speaking. When I joined PEERS, I was very shy, and it was hard for me to express my opinion. Now I am not as shy, and I can speak in front of an audience.

Last year alone PEERS conducted 67 presentations in the community. We also went on field trips to help our personal development. Terrific PEERS visited Lifelink, an organization run by persons living with AIDS, D.C. Hospital's boarder babies, the CADAC Drug Unit at St. Elizabeth Hospital, and the Walter Reed Medical Museum, to name a few.

Teens and adults usually respond well to our presentation, and I think it is because we come across like we know what we are talking about and are not afraid to say what we know.

Programs like PEERS are important in the fight to reduce risky behaviors among teens. I think that the federal government could best serve the needs of adolescents by funding more programs and organizations to do creative education, focused on different types of risky behavior.

Also, the government could develop more comprehensive health care facilities for adolescents or at least have comprehensive components at existing clinics.

I know that I am only 15, but my experience says adults will have to try some new methods or possibly lose many of today's youth.

Thank you for your time. I will try to answer any questions, and I hope you have some which are not too hard.

[Prepared statement of Eleshia Ray follows:]

PREPARED STATEMENT OF ELESHIA RAY, PEER EDUCATORS AND YOUTH COORDINATOR, PEERS PROGRAM, TERRIFIC INC., WASHINGTON, DC

GOOD MORNING TO ALL THE MEMBERS OF THE SELECT COMMITTEE ON CHILDREN, YOUTH AND FAMILIES. I WOULD LIKE TO THANK CONGRESSWOMAN PATRICIA SCHROEDER FOR GIVING THE PEERS PROGRAM AN OPPORTUNITY TO BE HEARD.

MY NAME IS ELESHIA RAY I AM 15 YEARS OLD, AND THIS IS THE START OF MY SECOND YEAR WITH TERRIFIC PEERS. I KNOW YOU ARE THINKING "WHAT QUALIFIES HER TO BE AN AIDS EDUCATOR?" WELL, WE ALL RECEIVED BETWEEN 40-45 HOURS OF TRAINING, WHICH WE TAOOK OVER A PERIOD OF 5 SATURDAYS. I LEARNED ALL ABOUT HIV AND AIDS, TRANSMISSION, PREVENTION, TESTING, TEEN PREGNANCY, STD AND DRUG ABUSE. I LEARNED ABOUT PEER PRESSURE, GOOD DECISION MAKING SKILLS, SELF ESTEEM AND LEADERSHIP.

THE PROGRAM ALSO TAUGHT ME HOW TO PREPARE PRESENTATIONS AND DO PUBLIC SPEAKING. WHEN I JOINED PEERS I WAS VERY SHY AND IT WAS HARD FOR ME TO EXPRESS MY OPINION. NOW I'M NOT AS SHY AND I CAN SPEAK IN FROM OF AN AUDIENCE. LAST YEAR ALONE PEERS CONDUCTED 67 PRESENTATIONS IN THE COMMUNITY.

WE ALSO WENT ON FIELD TRIPS TO HELP OUR PERSONAL DEVELOPMENT. TERRIFIC PEERS VISITED LIFELINK AN ORGANITION RUN BY PLWA, D.C. GENERAL HOSPITAL'S BOARDER BABIES, THE CADAC DRUG UNIT AT ST. ELIZABETH HOSPITAL AND THE WALTER REED MEDICAL MUSEUM TO NAME A FEW.

TEENS AND ADULTS USUALLY RESPOND WELL TO OUR PRESENTATION AND I THINK IT IS BECAUSE WE COME ACROSS LIKE WE KNOW WHAT WE ARE TALKING ABOUT AND ARE NOT AFRAID TO SAY WHAT WE KNOW.

PROGRAMS LIKE PEERS ARE IMPORTANT IN THE FIGHT TO REDUCE RISKY BEHAVIORS AMONG TEENS. I THINK THAT THE FEDERAL GOVERNMENT COULD BETTER SERVE THE NEEDS OF ADOLESCENTS BY FUNDING MORE GROUPS AND ORGANIZATIONS TO DO CREATIVE EDUCATION PROGRAMS FOCUSED ON DIFFERENT TYPES OF RISKY BEHAVIOR. ALSO THE GOVERNMENT COULD DEVELOP MORE COMPREHENSIVE HEALTH CARE

FACILITIES AT EXISTING CLINICS. I REALIZE THAT I AM ONLY 15, BUT MY EXPERIENCE SAYS "ADULTS WIL HAVE TO TRY SOME NEW METHODS OR POSSIBLY LOSE MANY OF TODAY'S YOUTH." THANK YOU FOR YOUR TIME, I WILL TRY TO ANSWER ANY QUESTIONS AND I HOPE YOU HAVE SOME WHICH ARE NOT TOO HARD.

Chairwoman SCHROEDER. Thank you very much, and are you going to address the group next?

Ms. STROUD. Yes.

Chairwoman SCHROEDER. Okay. The floor is yours, and you might, again, pull the mike just as close as you can. This is a cavernous room that eats words.

Ms. STROUD. Okay. Let me begin by saying good morning to the members of the Select Committee on Children, Youth, and Families, and thank you to Chairwoman Patricia Schroeder for extending an invitation to the Prevention, Education, Enrichment, Risk Reduction Strategies Program to be a part of these proceedings.

My name is Kianga Stroud, and I have lived in Washington, D.C. all of my life. As a teenager, I am concerned about the health and well-being of other teens.

I initially became involved with Terrific PEERS Program because I saw teens becoming infected with the HIV virus at a rapid rate. I was 13 at the time. I am now 15. So you can see I have been educating my peers for a while.

I realize that each of you is interested in hearing about the role PEERS educators play and whether we are accepted in that role. Our program, Terrific PEERS, believes that teens educating teens about AIDS is effective, and we strongly recommend it as one method.

PEERS has reached upwards of 10,000 people through radio, cable and community presentations. We go to teens wherever they are, whether it is their school; we go to their churches; the neighborhood recreation centers, as well as their summer job sites.

PEERS has also conducted presentations at the District STD Clinic.

As educators, we try to influence adolescent decisions regarding health issues. We demonstrate to our peers how a lot of their behaviors are unhealthy and can lead to AIDS and, finally, to death.

We communicate our message through role plays, videos, rap and straight talk. I believe the message is better received by the teens we are trying to educate because we are teens also, not adults. We are on the same level.

Also, our peers are impressed that we have so much information to offer and are able to articulate it.

I never participated in sex, drugs or any other risky behaviors, but PEERS has helped me to make the decision to continue to abstain from risky behaviors, and Terrific PEERS has truly helped me to increase my confidence and self-esteem.

In closing, let me say adults usually think they have all of the answers, but sometimes that is not true. So give the youth a chance to help with the answers.

Thank you, and I will try to answer any questions you may have.

[Prepared statement of Kianga Stroud follows:]

PREPARED STATEMENT OF KIANGA STROUD, PEER EDUCATORS AND YOUTH COORDINATOR, PEERS PROGRAM, TERRIFIC INC., WASHINGTON, DC

LET ME BEGIN BY SAYING GOOD MORNING TO THE MEMBERS OF THE SELECT COMMITTEE ON CHILDREN, YOUTH AND FAMILIES AND THANK YOU TO CHAIRWOMAN PATRICIA SCHROEDER FOR EXTENDING AN INVITATION TO THE PREVENTION EDUCATION ENRICHMENT RISK-REDUCTION STRATEGIES PROGRAM TO BE A PART OF THESE PROCEEDINGS.

MY NAME IS KIANGA STROUD AND I HAVE LIVED IN WASHINGTON, D.C. ALL OF MY LIFE. AS A TEENAGER I AM CONCERNED ABOUT THE HEALTH AND WELL BEING OF OTHER TEENS. I INITIALLY BECAME INVOLVED WITH TERRIFIC, INC.'S PEERS PROGRAM BECAUSE I SAW TEENS BECOMING INFECTED WITH THE HIV VIRUS AT A RAGPID RATE. I WAS 13 AT THE TIME, I'M NOW 15 SO YOU CAN SEE I'VE BEEN EDUCATING MY PEERS FOR A WHILE. I REALIZE THAT EACH OF YOU IS INTERESTED IN HEARING ABOUT THE ROLE PEERS EDUCATORS PLAY AND WHETHER WE ARE EFFECTIVE IN THAT ROLE.

OUR PROGRAM TERRIFIC PEERS BELIEVES THAT TEENS EDUCATING TEENS ABOUT AIDS IS EFFECTIVE AND WE STRONGLY RECOMMEND IT AS ONE METHOD. PEERS HAS REACHED UPWARDS OF 10,000 PEOPLE THROUGH RADIO, CABLE AND COMMUNITY PRESENTATIONS. WE GO TO TEENS WHEREVER THEY ARE, AT SCHOOL, TO CHURCHES, THEIR NEIGHBORHOOD RECREATION CENTERS AS WELL AS TO THEIR SUMMER JOB SITES.

PEERS HAS ALSO CONDUCTED PRESENTATIONS AT THE DISTRICT'S STD CLINICS. AS EDUCATORS WE TRY TO INFLUENCE ADOLESCENT DECISIONS REGARDING HEALTH ISSUES. WE DEMONSTRATE TO OUR PEERS HOW ALOT OF THEIR BEHAVIORS ARE UNHEALTHY AND CAN LEAD TO AIDS AND FINALLY TO DEATH.

WE COMMUNICATE OUR MESSAGE THROUGH ROLE PLAYS, VIDEOS, RAPS AND STRAIGHT TALK. I BELIEVE THE MESSAGE IS BETTER RECEIVED BY THE TEENS WE ARE TRYING TO EDUCATE BECAUSE WE ARE TEENS ALSO, NOT ADULTS. WE ARE ON THE SAME LEVEL. ALSO OUR PEERS ARE IMPRESSED THAT WE HAVE SO MUCH INFORMATION TO SHARE AND ARE ABLE TO ARTICULATE IT.

I NEVER PARTICIPATED IN SEX, DRUGS OR ANY OTHER RISKY BEHAVIORS BUT PEERS HAS HELPED ME TO MAKE THE DECISION TO CONTINUE TO ABSTAIN FROM RISKY BEHAVIOR AND TERRIFIC PEERS HAS TRULY HELPED ME TO INCREASE MY CONFIDENCE AND SELF ESTEEM.

IN CLOSING, LET ME SAY "ADULTS USUALLY THINK THEY HAVE ALL THE ANSWERS, BUT SOMETIMES THAT IS NOT TRUE. SO GIVE THE YOUTH A CHANCE TO HELP WITH THE ANSWERS." THANK YOU AND I WILL TRY TO ANSWER ANY QUESTIONS YOU MAY HAVE.

Chairwoman SCHROEDER. Thank you very, very much. We appreciated that.

And you are the one who taught them all, right?

Ms. TOURE. Well, yes.

Chairwoman SCHROEDER. Absolutely. Well, go for it.

Ms. TOURE. But it was not difficult.

I want to first say good morning to the committee members and observers, and thank you for the opportunity to appear before this committee as both a parent and director of a youth program focused on addressing risky behaviors.

Terrific, Inc. and Grandma's House developed PEERS as a means of reaching out to youth, offering them prevention education. It is clear that many of today's youth are involved in various kinds of risky behaviors: drugs, sex, alcohol, and negative peer pressure. Parents cannot begin to combat these behaviors without first realizing that their children may be at risk even if they are part of the ideal American Dream families like the Nelsons and the Huxtables.

The influences which exist outside the family are very strong. We live in an information age. If our children do not get the information from us, they will get it from other sources which may not necessarily reflect our values or our points of view.

Parents have to be willing to talk with their children about sex, drugs, AIDS, decision-making, and anything else which may affect their behavior and their safety.

Parents have to also be prepared to answer the hard questions with honesty and with courage, begin to share information at an early age, and as they grow, we can increase the amount of information we share, as well as the ways in which we share it.

To do this, parents must be comfortable with discussing these topics because it is important not to convey to your children that there is something wrong or that they are wrong to come to you. If you are uncomfortable as a parent with this role, what can you do?

First, you can discuss it with each other as parents, role play what you will say and how you will say it.

Seek out up-to-date information and familiarize yourself with it. Be aware of the current debates.

Do not isolate yourself. Talk to other parents. Find out how they are handling it.

Be prepared to listen, and please be open. Do not act surprised at what they say or how they say it. Keep in mind that as parents, we give our children morals and values, but they must make them work in today's world. We cannot do this for them.

Some of their perspectives will be different because their experience and their frame of reference is different, just as ours was somewhat different from our parents.

The idea that talking about certain behaviors will encourage you to participate in these behaviors is, in my opinion, dangerous. Not knowing all the facts seems more like it will make young people curious. Not being open makes them wonder what is the big deal, and it makes them more determined to find out and to know about it.

Finally, in terms of prevention activities for so-called minority youth, I believe that the best, most effective way to develop such programs would be to bring together frontline people already working with youth and allow them to come up with approaches and programs.

Also, in bringing youth together as a group, it would be important to include youth who have, in fact, benefitted from such programs and thus have had an opportunity to experience a change in their behaviors and a change in their attitudes. I believe that this will prove more effective than blue ribbon panels and ivory tower researchers.

Additionally, I would like to add that economic opportunities and prevailing social conditions will always be factors impacting the realities and, thus, the behavior of so-called minority youth.

We are products of our environment, each of us. It can be an environment with hope or one without hope, and each of you has the power to help determine that.

Thank you.

[Prepared statement of Nkenge Toure follows:]

PREPARED STATEMENT OF NKENGE TOURE, PEER EDUCATORS AND YOUTH COORDINATOR, PEERS PROGRAM, TERRIFIC INC., WASHINGTON, DC

GOOD MORNING COMMITTEE MEMBERS AND OBSERVES, THANK YOU FOR THE OPPORTUNITY TO APPEAR BEFORE THIS COMMITTEE AS BOTH A PARENT AND DIRECTOR OF A YOUTH PROGRAM FOCUSED ON ADDRESSING RISKY BEHAVIORS. TERRIFIC, INC. AND GRANDMA'S HOUSE DEVELOPED PEERS AS A MEANS OF REACHING OUT TO YOUTH; OFFERING THEM PREVENTION EDUCATION.

IT IS CLEAR THAT MANY OF TODAY'S YOUTH ARE INVOLVED IN VARIOUS KINDS OF RISKY BEHAVIOR DRUG, SEX, ALCOHOL AND NEGATIVE PEER PRESSURE. PARENTS CAN NOT BEGIN TO COMBAT THESE BEHAVIORS WITHOUT FIRST REALIZING THAT THEIR CHILDREN MAY BE AT RISK EVEN IF THEY ARE A PART OF THE IDEAL AMERICAN DREAM FAMILIES LIKE THE NELSONS AND THE HUXABLES.

THE INFLUENCES WHICH EXIST OUTSIDE THE FAMILY ARE STRONG. WE LIVE IN AN INFORMATION AGE IF OUR CHILDREN DON'T GET THE INFORMATION FROM US THEY WILL GET IT FROM OTHER SOURCES, WHICH MAY NOT NECESSARILY REFLECT OUR VALUES OR POINT OF VIEW. PARENTS HAVE TO BE WILLING TO TALK WITH THEIR CHILDREN ABOUT SEX, DRUGS, AIDS, DECISION MAKING AND ANYTHING ELSE WHICH MAY EFFECT THEIR BEHAVIOR, SAFETY, ETC. PARENTS HAVE TO ALSO BE PREPARED TO ANSWER THE HARD QUESTIONS WITH HONESTY AND COURAGE.

BEGIN TO SHARE INFORMATION AT AN EARLY AGE AND AS THEY GROW WE CAN INCREASE THE AMOUNT OF INFORMATION WE SHARE AS WELL AS THEY WAYS IN WHICH WE SHARE IT. TO DO THIS PARENTS MUST BE COMFORTABLE WITH DISCUSSING THESE TOPICS BECAUSE IT IS IMPORTANT NOT TO CONVEY TO YOUR CHILDREN THAT THERE IS SOMETHING WRONG OR THAT THEY WERE WRONG TO COME TO YOU.

IF YOU ARE UNCOMFORTABLE AS A PARENT WHAT CAN YOU DO? FIRST DISCUSS IT AS PARENTS, ROLE PLAY WHAT YOU WILL SAY AND HOW YOU WILL SAY IT. SEEK OUT UP TO DATE INFORMATION AND FAMILIARIZE YOURSELF WITH IT. DON'T ISOLATE TALK TO OTHER PARENTS FIND OUT HOW THEY ARE HANDLING IT.

BE PREPARED TO LISTEN AND BE OPEN, DON'T ACT SUPRISED AT WHAT THEY SAY OR HOW THEY SAY IT. KEEP IN MIND THAT AS PARENS WE GIVE OUR CHILDREN MORALES AND VALUES, BUT THEY MUST MAKE THEM WORK IN TODAY'S WORLD. WE CAN NOT DO THAT FOR THEM. SOME OF THEIR PERSPECTIVE WILL BE DIFFERENT BECAUSE THEIR EXPERIENCE AND FRAME OF REFERENCE IS DIFFERENT.

THE IDEA THAT TALKING ABOUT CERTAIN BEHAVIORS WILL ENCOURAGE THEM TO PARTICIPATE THESE BEHAVIORS IS IN MY OPINION DANGEROUS. NOT KNOWING ALL THE FACTS SEEMS LIKE IT MIGHT MAKE YOUNG PEOPLE MORE CURIOUS, NOT BEING OPEN MAKES THEM WONDER "WHAT IS THE BIG DEAL" AND IT MAKE THEM MORE DETERMINED TO KNOW ABOUT IT.

FINALLY, IN TERMS OF PREVENTION ACTIVITIES FOR SO CALLED MINORITY YOUTH, I BELIEVE THAT THE BEST MOST EFFECTIVE WAY TO DEVELOP SUCH PROGRAMS WOULD BE TO BRING TOGETHER FRONTLINE PEOPLE ALREADY WORKING WITH YOUTH AND ALLOW THEM TO COME UP WITH APPROACHES AND PROGRAMS.

ALSO IN BRINGING TOGETHER SUCH A GROUP IT WOULD BE IMPORTANT TO INCLUDE WHO HAVE WORKED IN SUCH PROGRAM AND YOUTH WHO HAVE BENEFITED FROM SUCH PEROGRAMS, THUS EXPERIENCING A CHANGE IN THEIR ATTITUDES AND BEHAVIORS. THIS WILL PROVE MORE EFFECTIVE THAN BLUE RIBBON PANELS AND IVY TOWER RESEARCHES.

Chairwoman SCHROEDER. Thank you very much, and I want to thank the three of you for coming.

One of the things I continually run into that amazes me is people tell me that even when they meet and talk to the parents about how important this communication is with young people, there are still a lot of them that just are not able to do it.

Do you encounter that? And what do you do? I mean are you able to have them break through some of that? What do you find are the biggest inhibitors in parents when it comes to this kind of communication?

Ms. TOURE. My experience is that a lot of it is fear. Before I worked with PEERS, I worked as director for community education at the D.C. Rape Crisis Center for 13 years, and we have done programs in the D.C. public schools around child sexual abuse, and from that experience and leading into this, I have found that a lot of parents are just fearful of discussing these topics, and I find that a lot of their fear is based on their being uncomfortable, not having the information at hand themselves, being unclear in terms of what their actual opinion or their feelings are regarding certain topics.

So it makes it very difficult for them to be able to convey that information when they have not resolved many of these issues themselves. I mean certainly if we think about sex, we can think about how it was for ourselves and how it was for our parents and how uncomfortable it was a lot of the time to talk about it.

So I think that parents have to educate themselves and be able to move beyond feeling uncomfortable, and they certainly have to move away from the idea that if they can somehow shut the information out and keep the information from their children, that their children will not be curious and will not seek it out because if they do not get the information directly from their parents, they will get it from their peers. They will get it from TV. They will get it some place.

Chairwoman SCHROEDER. That is what I have always felt.

What about the young people? Do you find you can work with kids to bring this up with their parents? Are there ways to get young people to be able to approach this with their parents?

Ms. RAY. Well, they could get information to share with their parents and explain it, educate themselves so that they can educate their adults.

Chairwoman SCHROEDER. And do you find that they do that or is there any way to know?

Ms. RAY. I really don't know. The presentations that we have, it seems as though maybe the students, the way that they accept it, that they may pass it on to peers and their adult parents, but there is no way of really knowing.

Chairwoman SCHROEDER. Congressman Wolf, do you have any questions?

Mr. WOLF. No, I do not, but let me just say something for the record. I apologize for not being here. I just do want to publicly state something with regard to witnesses.

I would like to request the chair if Mercedes Wilson could testify and for the following reasons. She is a Spanish witness originally from Guatemala who has been a Title 20 grantee and has evaluation data. This has nothing to do with this witness, but I think that the minority wants to protect its rights to have this witness testify because the minority has been faithful in attending these hearings. The minority has been faithful in participating. You have been faithful in being fair, and I would hate to see us break the balance and equilibrium that we have had.

As the Ranking Minority Member, I am just not going to develop a minority mentality. I have been here for ten years. The minority has a right to have a witness. We are going to have a witness. If we do not have a witness, then it will really be unfair.

So I would publicly like to request the Chair if we could have Ms. Wilson testify.

Chairwoman SCHROEDER. Well, I thank the gentleman. As you know, she has written testimony. We are more than happy to accept it for the record. Our problem is we did not hear about this until yesterday, and we had already thrown witnesses off because we have got such a busy morning, and there is a new member being sworn in.

The chair sat in the chair for over three and a half hours yesterday. Had we known before yesterday, we would have been more than happy to have had verbal testimony, but the record, and I would like to announce this for everyone, the record is open for two weeks. We would be very happy to accept testimony from people, and I am sorry that we did not know about this ahead of time, but time is moving along.

We have tried to be very fair, and most of these witnesses I do not think are coming with any political bent. I do not think we want to polarize this committee. They are coming talking as young people and parents about what they are trying to do, and I know there are very many others who would like to come.

We have had all sorts of people contact us, too, and I know each of you probably have people in your districts that would like to add things.

Mr. WOLF. Well, reclaiming my time though, I would tell the Chair that we were short one witness yesterday. This is not a political thing. The witnesses have all been good, and I commend them, but, under the rule, the minority has the right to call these witnesses.

Also, our witnesses, I have noticed, and I am sure it is just a coincidence, have in some cases been last, and in order to maintain the comity of this committee, which has been good, and I commend the chair, and I regret to raise this, but as the Ranking Minority Member, I have seen Minority Ranking Members who have allowed their rights to be trampled, and I will not do that.

Mr. DURBIN. Madam Chair.

Chairwoman SCHROEDER. Well, let me say——

Mr. WOLF. I just say I urge strongly that she be permitted to come, submit her statement, let the members look at it, and then answer any questions.

Mr. DURBIN. Madam Chair.

Chairwoman SCHROEDER. Let me say that the chair does not trample people's rights, and if the minority prefers having minority witnesses first on a panel rather than last, we would be happy to do that. We thought they wanted to be last to respond to other witnesses, and that that was the best position, but you know, we are not trying to be confrontational. We just cannot have people walk in when we have got witnesses backed up, and we have got all sorts of members here, and we know there is going to be a vote at 12:02 to do this.

Mr. DURBIN. Madam Chair.

Chairwoman SCHROEDER. The gentleman from Illinois.

Mr. DURBIN. If the gentlelady would yield, I think there are witnesses. I think this is an important issue that should be resolved within the committee structure perhaps when the witnesses are not present and we could have a meeting and agreement on a procedure.

These people have been kind enough to join us this morning, and a lot of us have other things we have to run to.

Mr. WOLF. Well, Dick, I have been at every hearing that we have had, and I am going to protect the rights of the minority.

Mr. DURBIN. I think you should.

Mr. WOLF. And I am prepared to talk about it publicly or privately.

Mr. DURBIN. Well, I hope you will.

Mr. WOLF. And if you do not raise these things, then the next person comes, and the problem occurs again, Dick.

Mr. DURBIN. I do not quarrel with your fairness.

Mr. WOLF. But I just want to make the point as an——

Mr. DURBIN. I am just quarreling with the timing this morning.

Mr. WOLF. But I want to raise it publicly so that it is out there——

Mr. DURBIN. It has been raised.

Mr. WOLF [continuing]. And people know. It has been raised, and if it is not addressed, it will continue to be raised.

Chairwoman SCHROEDER. And we will be more than happy to take her testimony as written testimony. As I say, I do not think we are going to have time for anything else.

The gentleman from Illinois.

Mr. HASTERT. Well, Madam Chair, I just have to look at this, too, and you know, you try and be fair, and we are in the minority, but I think we do make a contribution to this committee.

You know, yesterday your side added a witness at the last minute, and we were denied that privilege.

Chairwoman SCHROEDER. Not that I am aware of.

Mr. HASTERT. Well, look at the record. It happened, and you know, if you want to be fair and even-handed——

Chairwoman SCHROEDER. If it happened, it certainly did not happen with the chair's knowledge because that is not the rules of the procedure, and as I say, the chair was there, and many other members were not there for the full three and a half hours.

Now, I want to focus on adolescents in this society and their problems, and we can deal with these other things, and I am sorry, but——

Mr. WOLF. Well, it is not other things. We want to focus on adolescents and their problems, too, Madam Chair, but what we would also like to be able to have an across-the-board and an open dialogue here.

Chairwoman SCHROEDER. We are trying very hard to have that, and if you have some complaints about that, we will be more than happy to negotiate that and work that out. We have been bending over backwards to do whatever we could to do that, but I think what we want to do is proceed on and not waste any more of the witnesses' time, and we can work forward in the future to figure out what to do.

Is there anyone who has questions of this panel that they would like to ask?

Congressman Rowland.

Mr. ROWLAND. Yes. I want to talk about a hearing that we had in Macon, Georgia yesterday on health and education for adolescents and teenagers. It is certainly really a problem, and I would like to ask the witnesses.

One of the problems that was focused upon yesterday was the teenage or adolescent mother who has a child that also becomes a teenage or adolescent mother, and that perpetuates itself and goes on. One of the witnesses that we had, who is black and is a principal of a high school there now, said that her grandmother was a teenage mother, but her mother managed to break that cycle and give her children a chance to get an education, and this lady had become the principal of a high school.

But it is an awfully difficult thing to do, she said, because they have these children as a way of increasing the money coming into the family. Now, I would like to ask you: do you perceive it being that way? Is that one of the reasons that teenagers and adolescents have children, to get more money coming into the family? Is that one of the motivating factors?

Ms. RAY. Well, some people it seems as though that is why they have children at a young age, but others, like it is a product of their environment. That is all they know. They have grown up around their mother who was a teenage mother. So they think that that is right. So they do it, and it continues until somebody reaches and tells them, you know, it is not right.

Then as far as taking the money, I do not really think that that is why. You know, receiving welfare, is that what you are discussing?

Mr. ROWLAND. Yes. You do not think that is the reason?

Ms. RAY. No, I do not. I think it's because they are a product of their environment, and they think that is right.

Mr. ROWLAND. How do you break that? I guess that is a question I am asking.

Ms. RAY. Well, speaking with them, going to the root of the problem, giving them information.

Mr. ROWLAND. Are other teenagers doing that? I believe that you said that teenagers need to have the chance to provide information about the way that behavior should be; that they do not listen to adults as much, but they listen to other teenagers more.

Ms. RAY. That is true because when adults speak to teens, it is in an authoritative way, and sometimes they do not listen. They listen, but they do not pay attention to what teenagers or children are saying.

So when people on their own level say it, it seems more real because you see from, you know, the same age group, and they think that way, and they say, "Oh, well, hey, maybe that is true."

Mr. ROWLAND. A process of education?

Ms. RAY. Excuse me?

Mr. ROWLAND. A process of education. A process of education, is that the way that you have to deal with it?

Ms. RAY. Yes.

Ms. STROUD. Or maybe not even teenagers, but maybe other teenage mothers talk to other teens ahead of time, before they even got into the situation of being pregnant, talked to them and let them know that it is not all that it is cracked up to be. It seems that they see that they are getting welfare or whatever; that if they are getting money, they are making it.

So if other teenage mothers talk to them ahead of time, maybe that could stop teenage pregnancy.

Mr. ROWLAND. Thank you.

Chairwoman SCHROEDER. A good point, yes.

Congressman Peterson.

Mr. PETERSON. I would like to follow up on that. We keep talking about the teenage mother. Obviously, then, we have teenage fathers, and how do we reach the male side of this equation?

If there is anybody that has to be educated in this process, in the development of respect and the responsibilities that go with being active sexually, it seems to be the male, and in your group, the PEERS group, for instance, how large is that group and how many males are participating in this group along with you?

Ms. TOURE. A couple of things. The peer group is about from any given time between 10 and 18. It varies. The group is about three years old now. Last summer was the summer we had the largest percentage of male participation, which was about five or six male youth, teens, and we felt that was very good, and we were very pleased.

However, what we found was that there were some problems. The lure of sports was a problem. Wanting to have actual, full-time paying jobs was also a problem. It seemed that males didn't have the same level of interest in doing this kind of educational work.

Now, I do some coalition things in conjunction with the Center for Population Options, which has a youth group, the Everyday Theater, the Weight Theater Group, and we have all experienced difficulties with retaining participation of males on an ongoing basis the way that young women seem to be drawn to and participate in the groups. That is the first thing.

The second thing in regard to male responsibility, when we do the presentations, one of the places that we do them is at group homes, and these are group homes where males reside. When we do the male group homes, we do a two-part presentation. The first part is focused primarily around AIDS and risky behaviors, and the second part is focused around male responsibility, which is a follow-up presentation, when we go back and we kind of role play around, "Would you really use the condom? What are the things that would keep you from using a condom or the things that would encourage you to use a condom?" And kind of try to explore things, like if a girl came and told you that she was pregnant, how would you respond. Would you immediately respond, "This is not my baby," or "you're having sexual relations with other people, too," or whatever, and really try to explore with them what keeps them from using a condom or what would encourage them to use a condom and what would be their responsibility in these kinds of situations.

Personally, I feel that it would be very effective if there was a group of young men or a predominantly male group that developed some role plays and things and a whole program that focused around male responsibility and took that out and challenged other young people.

I think also a part of the problem for young men is that somehow the idea of being abstinent or saying no or whatever makes you less macho, puts your true maleness in question, and it should not be that way, and I think that they need role models that can go out and challenge that, and they need young men who can explore that whole train of thought, and I think that is very essential.

There are a few videos. There is one called "Male Responsibility" out of Oregon that is a group of young African American males who are in a rap group with a group leader, and some of them have children; some do not; and some are considering becoming sexually active.

And they are talking about what that means, and they have a few rap songs or whatever, and it is very good. It is very good because it raises those issues.

However, I do not see a lot of that kind of information and that approach being used, and I think that is needed.

Mr. PETERSON. I agree. I think if we are going to break this cycle, we cannot just concentrate on the teenage mother. We are going to have to concentrate on that teenage father as well and break this wimp factor that you are speaking to to some degree because if we do not do that, we are just not ever going to achieve any breakthrough on what you are talking about.

So I appreciate your comments. Thank you very much.

Chairwoman SCHROEDER. Does anyone else have questions?

Congresswoman Collins.

Ms. COLLINS. Thank you, Madam Chair.

I have to say that Mr. Peterson is on the right track. In Michigan, when I was a state representative, I got passed the sex education, birth control legislation in response to Planned Parenthood's Alan Guttmacher Institute book, Eleven Million Teenagers. What can be done about the epidemic of adolescent pregnancy in the United States? Speaking of sexually-active teenagers, and the main reason I did that was because I felt that the teenage girls were getting their information from the teenage boys, who got theirs in the back room and in the alley.

Since then I have found that the teenage pregnancies have gone up, not down, in Michigan, but I also read in an article in maybe Time or Newsweek Magazine that the percentage of teenage pregnancies were not that much drastically different in the 1700's and in the 1800's. Of course, people got married much earlier in those days, but the raging hormones existed in those days as well as they do today.

But the difference, I think, was in the responsibility aspect of it. If a girl got pregnant, I guess automatically they were married. The girl and boy were married, and today's society does not have those same conditions of not just shotgun marriage, but because they wanted to get married.

I think that perhaps we need to zero in on the teenage father, on parental responsibility, and I do know that sometimes in our community it is macho to have a baby, but if somehow or other we could get across the message that it is not macho to have a baby unless you are taking care of the baby, it might be a big difference.

It would be very good if some programs could be instituted at an early age on male responsibility.

Ms. TOURE. I agree with that, and with all due respect, I do need to say here that I think that in instituting programs that would address the question of male responsibility, I think that for those programs to be effective, we would have to look at the whole attitude of males in regard to sex in this society, and that is somewhat difficult to do.

I mean it is like we zero in on a piece of something, a small piece of the picture, and want to address that, but very often it is doomed to failure unless we can look at the whole picture, and the whole picture from my perspective has a lot to do with the attitudes that males in our society have in regard to sex.

You tell daughters to, you know, close your legs, and you tell males to go out and sow their wild oats. So you already have an initial conflict going right from the very beginning.

The woman's status in society is often based on "is she a virgin or not". There is value in being a virgin, but if the guy sits in the locker room and says he is a virgin, then all the other guys are going to laugh at him. So, of course, he is going to lie and talk about, "Yeah, you know, I got," whatever, and, "Yeah, I had her and I had her and I had her."

So I think that we have to do a whole thing, a whole societal thing in terms of conveying attitudes that say that it is okay not to be sexually active at any given time if you choose not to be.

Ms. COLLINS. Madam Chair, finally, I think her points are well taken, and it seems almost insurmountable to think of changing all of society's attitudes about sex, male sex versus female sex. However, it can happen.

I remember the sexual revolution. Was that the 1970s? It kind of passed me by, but I think it was the 1970s, and I thought America would never get back on a morality track, and then we had these horrible diseases come about, herpes and AIDS, and, boy, there was a turn-around, I think, in that free sex mentality in America.

So I am not wishing any horrible diseases, but perhaps we could make it just as unpopular to have unsafe sex, you know, for teenagers as the diseases did for the adults.

Thank you.

Chairwoman SCHROEDER. A very important point, and I must say your wisdom is just amazing that you exude.

I think what the chair had better do is call up the next panel unless there is some emergency question because we are running out of time. Let me thank you very much, and the next panel that we have is a very distinguished group.

We have, first of all, Dr. Selverstone, who is the president of the board of directors of the Sex Information and Education Council of the United States from Westport, Connecticut; Gil Walker, who is a commissioner of the Chicago Housing Authority and the Midnight Basketball League. That is very exciting because we want to hear how you motivate your males, and he is accompanied by one of the players, Mr. Selph, and we are very happy to have the two of you here. Maybe you can answer some of the questions we were dealing with just a moment ago.

We have Dr. John Lyons, who is the associate professor of psychiatry, psychology and medicine at Northwestern University Medical School. We have Bronwyn Mayden, who is the executive director of the Governor's Council on Adolescent Pregnancy in Baltimore, Maryland, accompanied by Cathy Cardall, a parent of a member of the Teen Council Program, and Dr. Bradley Hayton, who is the public policy research manager of the Focus on The Family in Pomona, California.

We welcome this very, very distinguished panel this morning, and we will put all of your testimony in the record, and if each of you care to summarize that would be just fine.

So if we can, Dr. Selverstone, let us start with you.

STATEMENT OF ROBERT SELVERSTONE, PH.D., PRESIDENT, BOARD OF DIRECTORS, SIECUS, SEX INFORMATION AND EDUCATION COUNCIL OF THE UNITED STATES, WESTPORT, CT

Dr. Selverstone. Madam Chairwoman.

Chairwoman Schroeder. That is right. Microphones help. They are such an aggravation. You would think they could work something out. Thank you.

Dr. Selverstone. Madam Chairwoman and members of the select committee, I am grateful for your invitation to be here. My name is Bob Selverstone. I'm a psychologist in private practice. I work with adolescents and with adult couples who are struggling in their relationships, and also with individual adults.

I have also been a teacher in the public schools for 30 years, starting in Brooklyn, New York, and for the last 25 years have been in Connecticut working in the secondary schools.

Twenty years ago my school system asked me to become the Director of Human Relations and develop programs in drug education, alcohol education, family life and sex education, and human relations education, and indeed, for the last 15 years I have taught, actually co-taught, both a human sexuality class and a values class at Staples High School in Westport.

Each year I make between 50 and 75 presentations both to parents and groups of teachers, but predominantly to groups of parents who are asking for help in dealing with communication with their children, their children's self-esteem, and issues of sexuality.

I am currently president of the board of directors of SIECUS, Sex Information and Education Council of the United States.

I think what I would like to do is address most directly the issue, Madam Chairwoman, that you raised in terms of how parents can be most effective. SIECUS' mission statement is that we will support the sexual rights of all people and collect and disseminate information about sexuality and support comprehensive sexuality education in the nation.

I think for most of us as parents, our view of reality is our projection from our own experience; that most of us grew up in a world in which sexuality was handled quite differently, and indeed, for most of the adult women in this audience, 20 percent had premarital intercourse, but indeed, 80 percent waited until they were married before having sex.

Currently it is exactly the opposite. Eighty percent of women have had sexual intercourse before they get married, and so it's very difficult for us as parents who know what our experience is, to understand that young people are going through an experience that is rather different from that.

When I ask parents what was the prevailing sexual climate and attitude as you grew up, and compare and contrast that with the sexual climate and attitude as young people are growing up, they recognize that there are both advantages now and also significant drawbacks.

And when I ask them if they would like their children's sexuality education to be a repeat of their own, they grimace and say, "Heaven help us. There has got to be a better way than the way that I learned about it."

Indeed, so many parents want help in sexuality education that the Harris Poll reports it is between 85 and 90 percent of parents who agree that there should be sexuality education in the United States.

Last year SIECUS published a booklet called Sex Ed. 2000, saying by the year 2000 all children should receive comprehensive sexuality education from pre-school through adulthood. Over 43 organizations have signed onto that goal, including the American Medical Association, the American Nurses Association, the American School Health Association, Children's Defense Fund, Girls, Inc., YWCA, and so forth. They are like most groups in the United States who really see this as essential.

Well, then the question is: how do we go about helping parents provide sexuality education for their children? SIECUS believes, indeed, I think with most people in the nation, that parents are and ought to be the primary sex educators of their own children.

Periodically people talk about school-based or youth serving agency-based or religious congregation-based sexuality education, and ask: "don't parents have the right to be the sexuality educators of their children?" and our answer is, no, they don't have the right; they have the obligation, which is far more powerful than the right.

And what parents are saying is that "we know we're not doing a good enough job, please help us." Even if I were, indeed, the world's best parental sex educator, and in the sanctity of the drawing room shared with my child the mystery and delight of sexuality, I would ill prepare my child for going out and dealing with his or her sexuality in the world because, indeed, they need experience talking about sex with peers because, indeed, that's where sexuality takes place.

I do three kinds of programs involving parents. At the end of our regular high school course we invariably say to our students, "You must bring your parents in for a two-hour evening session so that they will see the kinds of things that we talk about."

And at the end of that two-hour session, which is highly interactive, the parents invariably say, "Thank heavens, my children are experiencing this. I wish I did when I was their age."

It seems to me that the hurdles that get in the way of parents talking about sex are three or fourfold. I think for most of us there seems to be a natural reticence in thinking about our youngsters being sexual. I certainly remember diapering my son and daughter, and to imagine that that little bottom is going to be looked at and touched by someone else, I think, triggers a natural discomfort.

I think it is the same kind of discomfort that is triggered when children or even adults try to think about our own parents as sexual people. I suspect that is very difficult even for us in this room.

I think part of the reason why it is difficult—and one of the ways to get over it—is that parents' own sex education was inadequate, and I think what we need to do is to help reassure parents that they can learn. One of the real advantages in 1991 versus 1941 and 1951 is we now have excellent sources of information. We know things that we did not know before.

I think a second discomfort has to do with language. The very language of sex is often referred to as "dirty words," and some words are so offensive that it is like somebody scraping their fingers along a chalkboard, and other words are so medical and sophisticated that most of us really do not understand them. So I think we need to develop a language that both adults and youth can communicate on.

I think one of the problems is parents fear value conflict, and I think what we need to do is to acknowledge that and to recognize that in such a pluralistic nation as ours, there are indeed lots of values, and that one of the goals of democracy is to help people become more tolerant of diversity, and certainly in terms of sexual ethics, there is lots of diversity, and I think we need to help people learn how to communicate about that.

And, finally, I think is the issue of privacy. For most of us sex is a very private matter, and I am intrigued that the group that performed before you today talked about "secrets"; that one of the problems with secrets is we all go around believing we are the only ones who think or fear this. As people can begin to talk about it, we recognize that it is not such a terrible thing.

I guess the final thing I would like to address is some of the differences between mothers and fathers as sexuality educators of children. The data tends to be that mothers are sex educators twice as frequently as fathers. When I do a PTA program in lots of communities, I applaud the five to seven fathers who come on top of the 30 to 70 mothers who arrive, and the data is that the only time that fathers are approached as sex educators as frequently as are mothers is when those are fathers who are nontraditional; that they do the laundry, they do the cooking, they do the caring of the children, and they are seen as less fearsome authority figures, and therefore, people who can be approached with questions and concerns.

And the final thing has to do with the fact that research has demonstrated for quite some time that when mothers talk with their sons and daughters about sex, those daughters very often postpone the initiation of coitus or sexual intercourse. However, when fathers talk with their sons about sexual intercourse, as was alluded by the last speaker, with some frequency those young men initiate sexual intercourse earlier, and I do think it has to do with a pervasive sexual ethic among some men who feel that it is macho to go out and to score, and I think the message that we need to share with people is that sexuality is more than just genitals. It is the way that we relate to people, how we feel about ourselves as men and women, and our ability to love and to care and to respect the dignity of other people.

Research on sex education that attempts to measure the impact of five lessons on reproductive biology and one or two hours of talk about birth control is irrelevant. I think comprehensive sexuality education has not been evaluated because it has rarely been tried.

Knowledge and information is essential, but it is insufficient. We need to acknowledge feelings and values and attitudes and provide an opportunity for young people to talk about that with each other, and we need to help people develop communications skills so that they can get more information and give it, so that they can express their feelings and hear the feelings of others, and learn to make decisions that are in their best interest and the interest of other people.

Thank you.

[Prepared statement of Robert Selverstone, Ph.D., follows:]

PREPARED STATEMENT OF ROBERT SELVERSTONE, PH.D., PRESIDENT, BOARD OF DIRECTORS, SIECUS (SEX INFORMATION AND EDUCATION COUNCIL OF THE UNITED STATES), WESTPORT, CT

Madam Chairwoman, Members of the Committee, my name is Dr. Robert Selverstone. I am the President of the Board of Directors of SIECUS, the Sex Information and Education Council of the U.S. I have been a high school teacher and counselor for thirty years, and for the past fifteen years have been co-teaching a Human Sexuality course in Westport, CT, which I helped develop with community representatives. For the past dozen years I have also worked as a psychotherapist with teenagers and families, in addition to individual adults and couples.

This work has led to my being invited to make presentations and conduct programs and workshops on issues of adolescent development, self-esteem, communication, teen leadership, values and human sexuality throughout the country. In the past 15 years I have conducted over 500 programs for groups from the Pacific Air Forces, the National Association of School Boards and the National Association of Student Councils to IOWA Public Television, Children's Television Workshop and innumerable programs for parents and professional groups of teachers and mental health workers. The Human Sexuality course whose development I headed was named in a report to the then U.S. Dept. of HEW as one of twenty exemplary such courses in the nation.

SIECUS is a national non-profit organization headquartered in NYC. Founded in 1964, our mission statement reads:

> SIECUS affirms that sexuality is a natural and healthy part of living and advocates the right of individuals to make responsible sexual choices. SIECUS develops, collects, and disseminates information and promotes comprehensive education about sexuality.

SIECUS affirms that parents are - and ought to be - the primary sexuality educators of their children. SIECUS supports efforts to help parents fulfill this important role. In addition, SIECUS encourages religious leaders, youth and community group leaders, and health and education professionals to play an important role in complementing and augmenting the sexuality education received at home. We believe that the task of assisting our children in learning about their sexuality is a difficult one. Too often people seek to dichotomize this issue by asking: "But don't parents have the right to be the sexuality educators of their own children?" SIECUS believe that parents have not only that right, they have that obligation.

In March 1990, SIECUS released a national report, Sex Education 2000, outlining 13 goals to assure that all children and youth receive comprehensive sexuality education by the year 2000. Goal 2 reads:

> By the year 2000, all parents will receive assistance in providing sexuality education for their child(ren).

"Parents are the first and primary sexuality educators of their children. Parents provide children with their first understandings of gender roles, relationships, and values, and their first sense of self-esteem and caring. Infants and toddlers receive this education when parents talk to them, dress them, show affection, play with them, and teach them the names of the parts of their body. Older children continue to learn as they develop relationships within their own family and observe the interactions around them. In this way, parents set the framework for all other sexuality education efforts. Most young people look to parents as their most important source of information about sexuality, and more than two-thirds of young people have talked with their families about sexual issues.

Eighty percent of parents agree that it is their responsibility to provide sexuality education to their children, yet few actually do so. Only 25% of adults in the U.S. report that they learned about sexuality from their mothers or fathers. More than 80% of parents say they would like help in providing this information to their children. Many parents report that they are uncomfortable discussing such explicit sexual issues as intercourse, masturbation, homosexuality, and orgasm with their children, and that they would welcome assistance in doing so. In fact, some of the very topics which parents feel are most important to discuss are the ones they most often avoid discussing with their children. Almost 90% of American parents want their children to receive sexuality education in school.

Specific Approaches and Strategies to Assist Parents

In the over 500 workshops and presentations which I have conducted for adult groups, on issues of communication, values, alcohol and drug abuse, self-esteem and sexuality, I share my perception that there are a variety of forms of what I refer to as dysfunctional adolescent (and adult) behavior. These include suicide, homicide, interpersonal exploitation and violence, eating disorders, precocious sexual involvement and adolescent pregnancy, sexually transmitted diseases (including HIV/AIDS), racism, sexism, underachievement, risky auto driving, sexual abuse and assault (including acquaintance rape). Adolescence is indeed a "risky business". That is the bad news. These behaviors can be conceptualized as "branches" on a "dysfunctional behavior tree". The good news is that they appear to stem from a common trunk and root source, and if we can understand what that is, we can then begin to change it. We can either continue to feed poison into the tree or begin to input more nurturing nutrients. Indeed we do not need to develop specific programs to deal with the multitude of specific problems.

I believe the common nutritional source for this "tree" lies in understanding the normal developmental tasks of adolescents, how contemporary society affects them, and the importance of the key component, developing, nurturing and enhancing self-esteem.

Accordingly, most workshops which I conduct focus on issues of values, communication and self-esteem. If I can give parents better understanding of the commonality of problems and some skills to intervene then we can go a distance toward helping "vaccinate" young people against the blossoming of most of those dysfunctions.

I wish to outline how this works in three programs I conduct which are designed to assist parents in helping their children become sexually healthy adults.

The first is simply a "one-shot" presentation to raise parental and community consciousness about the fact that there are resources available to help them deal with the challenges they face in helping their children learn about sexuality. When I ask parents to reflect back upon the prevailing sexual climate and attitudes when they grew up and to compare that with the prevailing sexual climate and attitudes as their children are growing up, it is easy to see that there are some important advantages now at the same time that there some important new problems. When I ask whether they felt that their own sexuality education was well done and whether they would like their children to experience it just as they did, there is invariably a resounding "NO"! I then urge that the parents and other members of the community have the important responsibility to develop appropriate responses to such a challenge and indicate that while the task is often difficult the rewards are significant.

The other two workshops involve both parents and adolescents together. They are designed not merely to raise awareness, but most importantly to de-mystify the process of family communication about sexuality and to provide a successful experience in communicating and enhancing self-esteem.

One takes place at the end of the elective 9 week (one school quarter) Human Sexuality course which I have co-taught at Staples High School in Westport, CT for the past dozen years. Our students bring their parents to school for a 2-hour evening session which we conduct just as we do any other class; that means putting a premium on active involvement and participation. Parents and students are urged to speak with other participants who are not members of their own family, since they have lots of time later to share within their own family. The results of this are invariably enormously satisfying to both students and parents. In excess of 90% of participants find the evening to be enormously productive. Since we establish "Ground Rules" which make the class a safe place to speak and to listen, people feel comfortable in discussing the important and sensitive issues which are presented. Through this exchange of ideas and points of view, students are enabled to better understand some adult ideas and perspectives, and adults come to gain greater appreciation for the thoughtfulness and maturity which these 11th and 12th graders bring to bear in considering their important relationships. Some of you may have seen a portion of this class which was filmed and broadcast on a cable television station as part of a program on how parents can help their children learn about sexuality.

Among the reactions of parents who were moved to write of their reactions to the class are these:

- "The tenor of the class, clearly established from its inception, was one of acceptance, tolerance and respect for one another and for the various ideas presented. Each person had the option to share his or her ideas about a topic, as he or she saw fit. As a parent and a professional who works with families and with children who have suffered the trauma of sexual molestation, I cannot impress upon you enough the importance of such classes. Far too many families do not have the knowledge or communication skills needed to discuss the issues that are covered in these classes. Last night I observed parents and teenagers learning those skills while developing confidence and learning about themselves and what is important to them in an accepting, caring environment. It is these same young people who will be better able to make informed decisions about their lives while putting into practice effective communication techniques."

- "What I experienced last night was so powerful, it left me with that wonderful feeling of hope and wholeness that washes over me at choice instants in my life. Kids and parents were sharing some of their feelings about sexuality, about values, about love and family. They were talking to one another, exploring the differences and similarities between peers, generations and sexes. My decision making support system when I was seventeen was the views of my other equally adolescent friends. We spoke in hushes on the telephone and behind locked doors in the corners of our rooms. My daughter speaks openly in a classroom with trained professionals, peers of both sexes, and, thank God, her mother."

The third approach has been with a number of school systems who call me in to run a 3-4 part program for parents and their middle school children. The first evening is an orientation just for parents so they can get an overview of the developmental issues, and what they can expect from me over the remaining sessions when they will attend with their children. I have conducted these programs for as few as 50 attendees, and as many as 200 each evening.

What the programs do is confront what I perceive to be those major barriers to parent child communication which I believe can be addressed in this brief intervention. One problem is that most of us lack an appropriate vocabulary for talking about sex. While some words are so technical they are understood primarily by medical professionals, other words (slang) often carry so much emotional baggage that many of us find them offensive. Both sets of words then frustrate, rather than encourage communication. The task is to help parents and children develop a workable vocabulary which is both understandable and not offensive.

A second barrier is that many parents suspect that their own sexuality education is so deficient that they will be embarrassed by their lack of knowledge. Here, the greater openness of contemporary society about sexual matters, and the consequent availability of information is a real ally. SIECUS has both its own materials and bibliographies which can help parents and their children acquire this information.*

A third barrier is that for almost all of us the matter of sexuality has been a private (if not an outright taboo) topic. I am able to help both parents and their children consider this issue of privacy vs openness in seeking a better understanding of a strategy which is most productive and effective for them.

A fourth barrier is that parents anticipate and often fear values conflicts and confrontations with their children. Some of the activities conducted in the workshop are specifically designed to help participants examine their values, how their values might have developed and how people can discuss value differences productively. I believe this is a crucial issue, for in a pluralistic democracy, one of the essential needs for the improvement and civilized conduct of our society is that all of us develop increased tolerance for people with different values.

Finally, the thread which ties all of this together is a focus on communication skills, helping people become better listeners and learning to express themselves more directly.

With greater access to accurate information, increased understanding of one's own values and those of others, and with the requisite communication skills, parents are far better equipped to help their children become what we all hope for - young people who are developing the capacity for making important decisions, decisions which will protect them, those with whom they develop friendships and relationships, and the community at large.

The most extensive formal evaluation was conducted by the John Read Middle School in Redding, CT in 1982 and '83. Combining all the evaluations from all of the evenings, these were the results:

Program was of value to parents:	95%
Program was of value to students:	97%
Program was well presented:	98%
Program was informative:	98%
Program was interesting:	99%

After those two years we stopped the formal evaluations.

POLICY RECOMMENDATIONS

The task of sexuality education is one in which parents are pleading for assistance. Indeed, there are a variety of resources which could be made available. Accordingly, SIECUS offers for your consideration these policy recommendations:

1. All children and youth must receive comprehensive K-12 sexuality education. In October 1991, SIECUS will be releasing national guidelines for sexuality education. We estimate that less than 10% of young people in America receive this type of education. SIECUS is pleased that we have been able to play a leadership role among the 43 organizations which have demonstrated their commitment to this goal by joining in the National Coalition to Support Sexuality Education. The membership includes the American Medical Association, Girls, Inc, National Urban League, National Education Association, Society for Adolescent Medicine.

2. There must be increased efforts to help parents provide family-centered sexuality education to their children. These efforts could include new resource materials for parents, courses and workshops for helping parents become better sexuality educators of their children, and programs designed for both parents and children together. Workplace programs could address the difficulty of attracting busy parents to evening programs, and specially

designed television programs and videos - available from libraries and video stores - might help supplement such efforts. Both the SIECUS staff and I personally have been working in each of these areas.

3. Teachers, religious leaders, and youth serving agency personnel must receive specialized training in helping parents become the sexuality educators of their children. These teachers need certain personal characteristics as well as specific training and experience.

4. SIECUS calls upon the Congress, the Department of Health and Human Services, and the Department of Education to develop Federal policies and programs to encourage and strengthen sexuality education and family life programs. There should be Federal funding for training, technical assistance, materials, evaluations, and demonstration projects. Further, such programs should be positive, behaviorally-based and should not be limited to addressing problems related to sexuality.

It is incongruous that for most of this century the Federal government played a major role in promoting sexuality education, and only in this past decade has the Federal government withdrawn from this important area of concern.

5. Federal agencies should channel categorical funds into enhancing sexuality education efforts. For example, the Title X Family Planning Act, the Title V Maternal and Child Health Programs, the comprehensive health education efforts of the Department of Education, and the Department of Labor's Youth 2000 initiative could all address the sexuality education needs of children and youth.

6. Each Department concerned with children and youth needs to develop initiatives in support of sexuality education. There is not a single Federal official with responsibility for sexuality education. Each Department should clearly designate personnel with responsibilities for sexuality education. SIECUS calls upon the Department of Education and Department of Health and Human Services to designate staff with responsibility for these areas.

Parents want and must have this information. You have a critical role to play. The potential rewards are enormous. Unfortunately, we already know what the penalties are for not doing it; they are all around us.

Thank you.

Respectfully submitted,
Robert Selverstone, Ph.D.
SIECUS, President
June 18, 1991

*SIECUS Publications

For Parents

- How to Talk to Your Children About AIDS.
- Como Hablar Con Sus Hijos Sobre el SIDA.
- Oh No! What do I do Now? Messages About Sexuality: How to Give Yours to Your Children.
- I Ay No! Que Hago Ahora?
- Talking With Your Child About Sexuality and Other Important Issues.
- Growing Up - an annotated bibliography.
- Children, Adolescents, and HIV/AIDS Education - an annotated bibliography.

In Sexuality Education

- Sex Education 2000: A Call to Action.
- Winning the Battle: Developing Support for Sexuality and HIV/AIDS Education.

Chairwoman SCHROEDER. Thank you very much. That was very thought provoking.

Mr. Walker, we look forward to hearing you and Mr. Selph. Since there has been some discussion of males and how you reach them, it sounds like you have found a way to do this. So we will be very happy to hear about your program.

STATEMENT OF GIL WALKER, COMMISSIONER, CHICAGO HOUSING AUTHORITY, THE MIDNIGHT BASKETBALL LEAGUE; ACCOMPANIED BY BURTRELL SELPH, PLAYER, CHICAGO, IL

Mr. WALKER. Thank you. Good morning. Of course, my name is Gil Walker, and I am the Commissioner of the Midnight Basketball League in Chicago, Illinois.

To honorable Members of the Select Committee on Children, Youth, and Families, I bring you greetings from our Chairman, Mr. Vince Lane.

We are honored to be here to testify in front of this particular committee. Mr. Lane is, as I said, the Chairman of Chicago Housing Authority. Since he has been the Chairman, he came in with a new ideology, if you will, a new direction, that is, that if he is going to turn around the conditions in public housing, he is going to have to shift his emphasis, shift his emphasis from buildings and mortar to people, people programs.

He happened to be in New York on a particular occasion and heard about this program in Glen Arden, Maryland, right here in a suburb of Washington, DC, called the Midnight Basketball League, and asked us to investigate it, and we did.

We found out that they were playing basketball between the hours of ten to two, those hours because those were the time that crime was most prevalent in the community, and bad things were happening at that time.

Of course, you know about all the problems that plague Chicago and other urban communities, the gang problems that are running rampant. In investigating this program, we thought it was something that could work in Chicago, but of course, we feel that we are a little more sophisticated in Chicago when it comes to basketball than they are in Glen Arden, Maryland. After all, we are the NBA champs and have Michael Jordan.

Chairwoman SCHROEDER. I know. I know. Here come the Bulls.

Mr. WALKER. We picked Rockwell Gardens and Henry Horner. You have to come to Rockwell to understand the conditions there. I mean the gangs have taken over the community. You could not even go in the buildings to collect rent or to make any type of repairs.

The Midnight Basketball Program is a structured, organized, sophisticated program. It is not a rehabilitative program. It is a preventive program for young men between the ages of 18 and 25.

What we did prior to going into that particular development, during this particular program, you have to do in any area prior to bringing some type of resources, some type of program in. You have to go in and talk to the people in the community, and we used the same concept that, of course, the President used before we went to the war in the Gulf. You have to bring all the warring factions to the table first and talk about methods of control or trying to take care of the problem.

We went into Rockwell and Horner, and we sat down, and we talked to these young men because these young men control that particular community, not the police department, not the Chicago Housing Authority, not the City of Chicago. They controlled those particular communities.

And we talked about bringing this new, innovative program to them. We wanted to get their sanctions not to give the gangs any credibility, but for the program to work, they had to sanction the program, and they said, "OK. If you're going to do this, we're going to give you an opportunity to."

What we did was we selected 116 young men. We had 400 young men to try out for the program, but what we did was we called a practice session at six o'clock in the morning. We called one at two o'clock in the morning, and by attrition, they eliminated themselves.

The reason why we used basketball is because basketball, and I make no bones about it, is a national sport of the targeted population we are trying to reach. I do not care where you put a basketball hoop, in the middle of the Mojave Desert, within five minutes somebody is going to be slam dunking basketballs. Such is the magnetism that draws basketball.

There cannot be any teaching. There cannot be any educating, any instructions, unless you get someone's attention. Basketball gets their attention.

As I said, we are very sophisticated. We knew that we could not just give them a tee shirt and roll out a basketball. So what we did is we mirrored the approach of the National Basketball Association, not because we want these guys to think or put any illusions in their head that they are going to hone their skills and get into the NBA, but the NBA represents the very best there is in basketball, and we wanted our program to represent the very best there is also.

So we came up with brand new uniforms, brand new gym shoes, socks. We give championship rings. We have a banquet, all being that we are trying not only to try to draw them into the program, but we are trying to raise their self-esteem.

I have heard testimony here about manhood. What we are trying to do is undergird manhood, redefine manhood, if you will. Basketball is just a hook. Once we get them into this program, now they have got to listen to the gospel according to Gil Walker and the rest of the individuals who work in the program.

You see, I have never met a successful athlete that did not have a sound value system. We have to go back to the days of when I began to play basketball, and that was you may not have a father in the home, but there are surrogate fathers out there, and you have just got to tell it like it is.

These guys are between the ages of 18 to 25, but for some reason they failed society or society has failed them. What we find is that we have captured their attention the same way we capture the attention of 12-year-olds. They love basketball. That is the discipline, and because we have that discipline, they are going to obey the rules and regulations of our particular program, and that turns over to the rules and regulations of society.

I am not a social scientist. I do not know why basketball transcends political barriers, economic and social barriers, but it does. We have members of different gang factions who are playing on the same team now. The nay-sayers in the community, especially the police department, said, "Between the hours of ten to two you've got these guys in these different colors. They're going to be killing each other even more so than they are now."

Quite the contrary happened. These guys, we put them on the same teams. Instead of shooting at each other now, they are passing the basketball to each other. It is a mystical phenomenon that is happening within the Chicago Housing Authority. It surely could be spread throughout the nation.

We have team sponsors again adapting this same philosophy or policy of the NBA. You may not own a team in the National Basketball Association, but for $2,000 you can own a team in the Midnight Basketball League, and the phone just jumped off the hook with people who wanted to sponsor teams.

Sponsors were on-hands sponsors. They did not just give their $2,000 and that was it. These sponsors brought these guys to their homes. They took them to plays. They took them to restaurants. They really adopted these ten young men, and I will tell you the response has just been overwhelming.

We have 116 young guys in the program. At this particular time, we have 73 that are full-time employed. At this particular time, fifty-four went back to school to either get their GED or further their college education.

Now, we are talking about individuals for the most part that used to rob and steal and snatch purses to survive out there. Because of this Midnight Basketball League, because we show them another alternative, because we are showing them even though you are between the ages of 18 and 25 and you are out there, there are some people in this society who still love and care about you. If you are willing, if you are willing to get involved in this program and take a chance on us, we are willing to take a chance on you.

So I repeat: this is not a rehabilitative program. If you mess up, once you are in this program, we will kick your behind out. This program is for guys who are not intent on doing criminal activity, but guys who may have done something in their past, but now who want to take the opportunity to turn their lives around. We are there for them.

We pay coaches. We pay officials. The program costs. It costs about $80,000 to put 116 young men through a 16-week program, but we keep hands on with them all year long.

I submit to you that the program is cost effective because, as you very well know, it takes about the same amount of money to incarcerate a young man for two years. Since the inception of the Midnight Basketball Program in Glen Arden, Maryland, and since the inception of the program in Chicago, not one young man, not one, has been incarcerated or been in trouble for any reason.

I could go on and on about this particular program, but time will not permit, but Burtrell Selph is here. He is a participant in the program, and I would like Burtrell to just give you some comments on how he feels about the program.

[Applause.]

Mr. SELPH. Hello. First of all, I would like to extend my gratitude for the invitation here to Washington, D.C., to Patricia Schroeder and the Select Committee on Children, Youth, and Families.

I am here to give a self-testimonial of what Midnight Basketball has done for me. It has given me a father figure and something to look forward to in a sport that I love, which is basketball, and it has given me most of all self-motivation.

I have also started back to school. I have a 3.0 grade point average. I work at the Chicago Mercantile Exchange. I am an R clerk, and if you have any questions, I will be happy to try to answer them, you know, after everything is over.

[Prepared statement of Gil Walker follows:]

Prepared Statement of Gil Walker, Commissioner, Chicago Housing Authority, Midnight Basketball League, Chicago, IL

INTRODUCTION AND OPENING

Hello:

My name is Gil Walker, Commissioner of the Chicago Housing Authority's Midnight Basketball League.

To the Honorable Members of the Select Committee on Children, Youth and Families, we bring to you greetings from our Chairman, Mr. Vincent Lane, as well as Chicago public housing residents, our departmental staff, and members of the Midnight Basketball League Family of supporters, participants and sponsors.

We are honored and pleased to be extended this opportunity to testify on how Midnight Basketball impacts on the lives of our youthful player participants.

BACKGROUND

G. Van Standifer was a City Manager for the town of Glenarden, Maryland struggling with the problem of escalating criminal and drug activity in the township, against considerable local opposition, implemented **Midnight Basketball** in Prince George's County in 1986. Games were played two nights each week from June until August. The following year, 1987, the city of Glenarden witnessed a significant decline in the number of crimes reported.

The Chicago Housing Authority's **Midnight Basketball League (MBL)** is a franchise of the established MBL in Prince George's County, Maryland.

The most significant individual directly responsible for our program being developed was the Chairman of the Chicago Housing Authority who had the vision and set a tone which stimulated support from other governmental agencies and private resources to become partners in this venture. The program has full support of the Superintendent of Police, in addition to various city service departments such as the Department of Health, Department of Human Services. More support arrived from the City College System, with the use of their facilities as well as the willingness to provide educational services to our players. Further the positive program exposure by various media professionals, such as George Wills, Curry Kilpatrick, Mike Gillis of the Chicago Sun Times has been a tremendous asset to this program.

PROGRAM DEFINITION

Midnight Basketball is a viable alternative to a lack of positive late night recreational options. The "hanging out," of young males from 17 to 25 years of age during the hours of 10 p.m. to 2 a.m. creates a climate which is conducive for negative activities, a notion confirmed by police statistics. Therefore, as part of a comprehensive anti-crime strategy, called Operation Clean Sweep, the Chicago Housing Authority has instituted the **Midnight Basketball** Concept within two public housing developments.

Midnight Basketball is unique in that it takes an old concept--sports as a constructive character building activity--and gives it a new twist - the organization of a structured program, "after hours." In addition to utilizing basketball as an attractive, off-the-street- activity, components have been added which are designed to encourage the participants to take charge of their own life, family and destiny, i.e., Employment Development and Training, Life Planning and Group Motivation, Mentoring and Support Services Network.

The goals of **Midnight Basketball** are as follows:

1) Provide and develop a comprehensive structured P.M. program which would result in a productive alternative to criminal activities for young male adults between ages 17 through 25;

2) Develop a mechanism for the identification and cultivation of natural alternative young adult leadership through the use of a sports medium;
3) Develop and provide a network and array of support services which will enhance and have a positive impact on the participants' quality of life; and
4) Provide a structured activity which was very intense as well as demanding of discipline and good character; thereby preparing participants for future opportunities.

MIDNIGHT BASKETBALL OPERATIONAL ASPECTS

The target population of **Midnight Basketball** are public housing males who reside within a designated public housing development. Participants are identified and recruited by three methods: (1) Referrals from community organizations, Resident Local Advisory Councils; (2) Word of mouth; (3) Departmental Outreach Efforts.

Selection is based on the ability and willingness to comply with all program guidelines. Further participants must submit to a security check.

A **Midnight Basketball** participant is generally: Unmarried African-American male who lives in public housing; Has 2 children between 2 to 5 years of age; is unemployed or underemployed;

Has tremendous influence among the youth within those targeted developments. Our clients are defined by geographics and age as well as gender. There are 6,435 residents within Henry Horner and 4,102 residents within Rockwell, the bulk of which are children and youth. This program serves directly 160 to 200 clients.

Midnight Basketball utilizes sports as the program nucleus upon which all other satellite activities revolve around. The use of basketball constitutes both a lure and hook to introduce program participants to other personally needed programmatic activities. Those satellite activities and functions are Life Management Workshops, Group Motivational Seminars, Support Services Component, Employment Development and Training.

(A) Life Management Workshops are mandatory team sessions designed to increase personal self-awareness as well as to develop inter-personal skills; these sessions are instructive and motivational in nature.

(B) Motivational Seminars - are mandatory for all league players. Such seminars are designed to change a player's outlook on life as well as to inspire attitudal changes. Further these seminars are conducted by various famous personages who provide some personal insights of their own lives, as well as how they handle such challenges. One such person was former boxing champion Buster Douglas, who later donated $10,000 to the program. Participants also interact with various sports celebrities and team sponsors.

(C) Support Services - these services range from counseling, educational services to mental health, depending on the participants' needs. Such services are available per a player's request. All players are encouraged to utilize these services.

(D) Employment Training and Development - this programmatic aspect is to assist those participants who desire employment to become job ready, as well as to secure employment for them through various program relationships and personal connections. This is one of the most crucial components.

CHA has presented a **Midnight Basketball** Program adaptation with flair, and style, but most crucial is the appeal it has with street youth. The program's psychology and marketing is to use prestige as a method of luring potential participants to the program. Big city youth are very sophisticated and want recognition as well as visibility; **Midnight Basketball** provides just that. Therefore, resources are expended on uniforms, gym shoes which are given to the players. Further, the CHA program is modeled around the National Basketball Association. The champions are given rings, banquets, etc.

The CHA program has paid staff, players' retreats. This year a new service contract between players and **Midnight Basketball** Program Management will be implemented. The agreement will outline what services are wanted and needed by the participants. This agreement further states staff's role in rendering assistance to the participant in accomplishing their personal goals.

The CHA **Midnight Basketball Program** runs year around rather than just during the summer months.

PROGRAM IMPACT

Midnight Basketball has enhanced the Authority's capacity to build collaborative relationships with other public and private sector entities. Further the positive public exposure has caused a strong response of community volunteers to participate in CHA sponsored programs. But the player-participants, have gained the most, for example, no player has been arrested, 41 have received employment, 54 are registered for classes at a local community college. Some participants have traveled to D.C. as a result of this program, as well as California to complete a movie. **Midnight Basketball** is presently at Rockwell Gardens and Henry Horner Homes. **Midnight Basketball** will expand into four other public housing developments during 1991 per popular demand. The three program standards of measurement are as follows:

1) Program Retention and Participation - only four of 160 players have dropped out from this program.
2) Criminal Involvement - thus far no players have been arrested, to do so would result in termination from this program.
3) Suspension - only four suspensions have occurred during 89 - 90 season.

By far, the strongest supporters of the League are its sponsors who provide tremendous resources as well as invest their time and energy into their team's development. Without this type of support, there would be no credible **Midnight Basketball League** within Chicago.

Our sponsors can be characterized as "investors in human capital." These team sponsors are generally businessmen who truly have scrutinized the program's bottom line..the development of young men into productive citizens. And therefore have committed themselves to assure the sussess of the League.

Midnight Basketball's greatest achievement is the tremendous hard-won support of its service population, the residents of public housing. This is the most popular program in CHA.

Such popularity has led to a high level of program demands. Further, this support brings great credibility to the Department, its staff and the Authority.

Midnight Basketball was evaluated by Dr. Walanga Kpo of Chicago State University for Windows of Opportunity, a non-profit corporation which was founded by the Chicago Housing Authority. The contact person for these materials is Ms. Sandra Harris, who can be contacted at (312) 791-4768, 534 East 37th Street, 1st floor. She would gladly send you a copy of the evaluation.

"The Program has accomplished its short-term goals. Further, the play participants who completed the program, reported increased self-esteem, acquisition of new skills, and self-development and educational and job opportunities. The most significant short-term success is the participants' perception that CHA Leadership cares about what happens to them. All coaches throught the program to be useful to participants. Sponsors believed the program to be useful, has great potential, should be expanded to include more CHA development residents. Sponsors believe this program investment to be an excellent one."

Today's youth are, indeed, tomorrow's adults. Children are our greatest national treasure. Without youth, a nation can not hope to have a lifeline for the future..for youth are the future to be.

If, indeed, it is truly believed, then this great nation must reflect that in its national policy and resource allocation. Clearly America must invest in its adolescenses, children.

One of our greatest challenges in working with so-called high risk youth is the lack of options and resources. We need more dollars for early intervention and prevention programing and models. We need a way of employment training youth to be economically viable, so that the selling of drugs is not an option. We need to know what works and what doesn't in intervention or prevention. What we do today will determine the type of future this nation is to have tomorrow.

Thank you for your concern.

[The Summary Evaluation Report: Midnight Basketball League Program 1989–90 Pilot, December 17, 1990, is retained in committee files.]

Executive Summary of Midnight Basketball League Program 1989–90 Pilot

Purpose
The purpose of this report is to evaluate the Midnight Basketball (MBL) program developed by the Chicago Housing Authority (CHA). The evaluation focused on the four objectives of the MBL program. The evaluation was focused along three perspectives, namely, MBL objectives, participants' perceptions, and third party stakeholders' (support service staff, sponsors, media) perceptions of the program. Information for the evaluation came from several sources - MBL program files, police crime statistics, surveys, interviews, sponsors, and news media. This information was used to determine the accomplishment of program objectives.

Findings
From the three evaluation perspectives the program accomplished its short-term objectives. Short-term outcomes included the provision of constructive divergence from socially unacceptable behaviors during the program period. Participants who completed the program refocused their ambitions to further education, employment, desisting from gang, criminal, and drug activity. Participants reported increased self-esteem, acquisition of new skills, self development, and, educational and job opportunities. Officially, success stories included one vocational training graduate, one GED graduate, 12 adult education completions, and 27 employments. Long-term objectives were too premature for evaluation at this time.

Probably the most significant short-term success is the perception of participants that the CHA leadership cared and was willing to give them a chance to avail themselves of opportunities in the real world. It is too early to evaluate the long-term effect of the program on objective criteria such as job retention, decline in verifiable criminal activities and, educational achievement.

All 16 MBL program coaches believed the program to be useful to participants, that it gave them new skills, self-esteem, and opportunities. They, however, recommended longer workshops and season for the program. Team and program sponsors believed the program was useful, has great potential, and should be expanded to include more CHA development residents. Their evaluations suggested that they had received a good return on their investments. News media perceptions were also favorable to the program. Program coverage touted the vision of the CHA leadership, potential of the program, and support for it. The news media has not made any evaluations of the program yet. In spite of agreement in perceptions, the following deficiencies were observed:

1. Inadequate individualized needs assessment and goal setting.
2. Lack of customized activities to meet participants needs.
3. Inadequate program monitoring and documentation.
4. Lack of formal service or training modules from service providers.

5. Lack of participant orientation in the importance of accuracy and completeness of personal program information.

In order to improve the long-term success of participants and the MBL program, the following recommendations are made in part to reduce the above program deficiencies. Some program improvement suggestions have also been made.

Recommendations:

1. Needs assessment and goal setting:
   Individual participant's needs should be assessed at the beginning of the program to identify personal needs within the realm of the MBL program capabilities - education, employment counseling, job readiness, drug counseling, vocational training, crime prevention etc. Based on the needs identified, personal goals should be set for individuals for the duration of the program. Participants should be trained in setting explicit and measurable goals that could be readily assessed.

2. Customized activities:
   In addition to common activities, individual participants should be engaged in activities that facilitate the achievement of their personalized goals.

3. Program and individual monitoring:
   Short-term program and individual objectives should be periodically monitored to ensure that activities are indeed contributing to targeted outcomes. This process also affords a short-term review of direction, focus and relevance of program activities to program goals, and facilitate revisions where appropriate. The short-term outcomes further serve as a source of motivation to participants when progress and feedback are immediate. Monitoring devices such as questionnaires or interviews should be developed for this purpose.

4. Service/training modules:
   Each service provider should explicitly indicate what services will be provided, the objectives of the service expected outcomes, and when and how outcomes would be evident. At the end of the service an evaluation should be conducted to see whether services were provided as proposed and whether the intended outcomes were evident. This would determine the need for further services in a given area. Questionnaires or interviews should be developed for this purpose.

5. Participant education/orientation:
   Participants should be briefly educated in the importance of providing accurate personal information, program evaluation, and the confidentiality of such information. They should also be instructed on how to complete all forms, thus preparing them to cope with the demands of contemporary society replete with information documentation.

6. Group incentives:
   Teams should be offered incentives for group achievements in education, keeping out of trouble, decreased drug use and criminal activity, attendance, program completion, number of certificates awarded, employment and social responsibility. Teams should come up with strategies to improve these accomplishments and also determine what incentives they prefer to be used as rewards for achievement. Teams should also be encouraged to collectively solve program-related problems with coaches and CHA personnel functioning as facilitators. This strategy should foster cooperation, responsibility, problem solving skills, perception of personal control, and define the path-goal relationship for their personal lives.

7. Longitudinal monitoring of successes:
   Participants who indicated they were planning to continue their education, who are employed, or still in school should be monitored closely to assess their progress. The MBL program should continue to provide whatever assistance possible to ensure participants' success at their chosen endeavors. For motivation, successful alumni should be encouraged to return as mentors to current program participants.

Chairwoman SCHROEDER. I want to say the gospel according to Gil Walker is very impressive. If we could only clone you. But I really want to thank you.

Let us move on to our next witness. I do not envy you, Dr. Lyons, having to follow that, but the floor is yours.

STATEMENT OF JOHN F. LYONS, PH.D., ASSOCIATE PROFESSOR OF PSYCHIATRY, PSYCHOLOGY, AND MEDICINE, NORTHWESTERN UNIVERSITY MEDICAL SCHOOL, CHICAGO, IL

Dr. LYONS. Yes, I was thinking the same thing.

I think though that there is a good point here, if I could mention it as an aside, for those of us who feel that we cannot teach values. I think Mr. Walker's program is an excellent example of how that particular problem can, in fact, be approached.

What I would like to spend some time testifying about, and I thank the committee and Madam Chairperson for the opportunity, is to talk a little bit about the other side of the problem: the school-based health clinic approach.

Since the school based health clinic first went open in Dallas in 1970, this type of theoretically comprehensive health care service delivery has been greeted with both considerable enthusiasm and skepticism.

Enthusiasm has stemmed from the potential these clinics have offered for meeting the acute and complex health needs of our nation's young people, particularly those in impoverished, usually urban environments, in which health care access has been limited.

My own Representative, Representative Collins, has been instrumental in the implementation of these programs.

Skepticism comes primarily from the focus of the school-based clinics on pregnancy prevention through contraception. This committee observed that while national rates of births to teenage parents declined from 1970 to 1982, pregnancy rates among teenagers nearly doubled. Teenage pregnancy rates continue to climb, particularly among unmarried adolescents.

Unfortunately, the debate about the utility of school-based health clinics has been drawn along partisan lines. Given these political considerations, it might be informative to pursue the question from a purely scientific perspective.

All parties would seemingly agree that teenage health is a major national concern. Likewise, all would agree that pregnancy represents a major threat to the lifelong wellbeing of teenagers, particular unmarried adolescent girls.

The policy issue then becomes: what is the best mechanism to address the problem? That is, how do we reduce the number of teenage pregnancies?

From a scientific perspective, the controversy over the role of school-based health clinics and pregnancy prevention can be reduced into a clearly addressable question. Do school-based clinic programs reduce the rate of pregnancy among the children and adolescents they serve? And if so, what are the characteristics of those programs that are most effective and those that are least effective?

Regardless of political persuasion or prior belief about the efficacy of these clinics, it is unlikely that the validity of posing this particular question is particularly controversial. However, answering this question through the use of existing empirical research represents an important challenge fraught with the potential for controversy.

Traditional reviews of the literature are often questioned, based on the selection of articles to be reviewed and different criteria used to evaluate one article and another. In order to review a literature in a fashion that cannot be criticized based on arbitrary decisions, the selection of articles and the criteria on which they are evaluated must be formally specified and reliably applied.

This technique of literature review first proposed by Light and Pillemer in 1984 is called systematic analysis. I, along with a number of colleagues, have used systematic analysis to study such issues as nursing home care, AIDS research, services for the seriously mentally ill, and the effects of aggressive pornography on violence towards women.

We have consistently found high reliability. The reliabilities of the reviews are invariably over .95, which basically means that anybody in this room could repeat the review in the same fashion that we did and find exactly the same results.

In order to study the efficacy of school-based clinics, we undertook a systematic analysis of the existing scientific literature. For the present analysis, a computerized Medline and PsychLit, two databases, search from 1976 to 1990 identified 100 articles on school-based clinics published in peer reviewed journals. Peer-reviewed journals are selected as a quality control because there is a lot higher standard of scientific efficacy for those articles than for reports and book chapters and unpublished documents.

Thirty-four of these 100, or 34 percent, were empirical studies in that they reported at least one summary numeric result. Nearly two-thirds of the articles were nonempirical and included literature reviews, commentaries and editorials. In general, that is not a very good showing in terms of the amount of evaluation research for a particular area, a relative to nursing home research.

The 30 empirical studies generally did not address the range of possible services proposed for school-based clinics. Rather, 26, or 76 percent, three-quarters, focused almost exclusively on pregnancy and contraception issues and services. Only five of these studies included any measures of other health concerns. Seven, or 21 percent, focused on prenatal or postnatal health services.

None of the studies investigated educational programs which emphasized abstinence as a form of pregnancy prevention, although several did study the effects of clinic operation on the onset and frequency of sexual behavior.

The absence of abstinence research is compared to 21 studies focusing on contraception, primarily condoms and birth control pills, and six studies concentrating on abortion.

One study investigated the role of adoption as an option in the resolution of unwanted pregnancy.

Eight of the 34 studies were retrospective or prospective evaluations of the impact of school-based clinic programs. In other words, those were the best. Six of these studied effects on sexual activity, contraception, pregnancy and/or birth rates, which are the four critical dependent variables in any pregnancy prevention research.

On these four critical variables, the results across studies can be summarized as follows. For sexual activity, there is little evidence that clinics reduce or delay sexual activity. In fact, no study reports a statistically significant decline in sexual activity.

On the other hand, there appears to be no consistent evidence that clinics stimulate more sexual activity. Only one of the studies had a higher level of sexual activity associated with clinic operation.

So on this dimension, the programs appear to be generally inert.

Contraception. There is fairly consistent evidence that clinics increase teenage access to contraceptives, primarily female teenagers, teenage girls. Clinics generally report fairly high utilization consistent with the testimony this morning. The utilization rates for males is much, much lower.

There is substantially less evidence to show that contraception provided by the clinics is used more often. This is usually measured by asking the teenager whether or not they used contraception at the time of last intercourse. There is only one study that has a statistically significant increase in the amount of times that contraception was used at the last intercourse.

So although there is consistently access to contraception, it does not appear that contraception is consistently used. Part of this problem may be that studies show that knowledge about contraception increases statistically significantly, but it does not become perfect. On average, across the studies students participating in the clinic programs move from about 70 percent of the time being right on questions about contraception to 80 percent of the time being right. So on a ten question test, the "before clinic" get seven out of the ten right; "after clinic" get eight out of the ten right.

For pregnancy, perhaps the most important, there is little consistent evidence that the clinic programs affect pregnancy rates one way or the other. There is one study that shows a statistically significant decline. Two studies report increases. In the remaining of the studies, the program appears to be inert.

For birth rates, there is fairly consistent evidence that school-based clinics do reduce birth rates. The mechanism for this effect, however, does not appear to be due to the reduction in pregnancy. Rather, birth rates appear to be reduced primarily through the use of abortion.

In summary, ideally a well-functioning school-based clinic should have a range of therapeutic services designed to meet the varying needs of school-aged children. These might include, among other services, immunization, vision and hearing screening and counseling services.

The scientific evaluation literature on these clinics, however, has clearly focused on the role in pregnancy prevention through contraception. There is data to suggest that contraception is, in fact, a main reason that students visit the clinics.

If clinics are providing other services, they generally do not appear in the scientific literature. There is one exception in 1989. A piece in Public Health Reports that evaluated a comprehensive health care program and found no effects on medical outcomes.

As I mentioned, school-based health clinics appear to have failed to meet their mandate. A good pregnancy prevention program should have the following outcomes.

Number one, a reduction in sexual activity and/or a reduction in the absolute number of unprotected sexual encounters.

Two, as a direct effect of outcome one, a reduction in the number of pregnancies. Primary prevention of pregnancy requires one of two things: either abstinence, no sexual activity, or contraception.

No published research has focused on the former. The latter does not appear to be clearly effective with teenagers.

It does not appear that school-based health clinics achieve their goal of primary pregnancy prevention. Secondary prevention would involve either abortion or adoption. It appears that some clinics achieve secondary prevention through the use of abortion. Adoption as a form of secondary prevention has received almost no study.

Although admittedly selected for their impact, three quotes from a recent study in *Family Planning Perspectives* by Kirby, Waszak and Ziegler in 1991 dramatize the problem.

First, "in sum, simply providing contraceptives was not enough to significantly increase their use."

Two, "analysis of post data from the San Francisco clinic revealed that females (not males) were significantly more likely to have sex than they had been before the clinic opened."

Three, "clinic presence was not associated with lower rates of pregnancy at any sites, either during the previous 12 months or at any other time. In Dallas, the proportion of females who reported they had ever been pregnant was higher at the clinic school than at the comparison school."

In discussing the findings, these authors were supportive of the clinic endeavors. However, their data, consistent with previous studies, portrays six school-based clinic programs as failing to meet their goals of pregnancy prevention.

The authors noted that those clinics with the larger educational programs that emphasize responsibility in sexual relations and follow-up care appeared to be somewhat more effective than the others. This observation is consistent with a recently published study by Howard and McCabe in 1990 reporting successful reductions in sexual activity through the use of an educational program that emphasized premarital sexual abstinence.

Teenage pregnancy is one of the greatest risks in the risky business of adolescence. When this committee decides how best to pursue the public policy to address this problem, I hope that you will consider the following.

One, school-based health clinics are relatively understudied, and the focus of the small amount of well-done research has been on contraceptive services. What other needs these clinics serve must also be studied along with the impact of any of those services.

Second, school based health clinics do not appear to be successful at reducing teenage pregnancy. Other approaches deserve study. Alternatives to these clinics, particularly educational programs that emphasize delay in sexual activity, have not received much research attention or funding.

Thank you.

[Prepared statement of John F. Lyons, Ph.D., follows:]

PREPARED STATEMENT OF JOHN F. LYONS, PH.D., ASSOCIATE PROFESSOR OF PSYCHIATRY, PSYCHOLOGY, AND MEDICINE, NORTHWESTERN UNIVERSITY MEDICAL SCHOOL, CHICAGO, IL

A Systematic Analysis of Research on the Impact of School Based Health Clinics

Since the first school based health clinic opened in Dallas in 1970, this type of health care service delivery has been greeted with both considerable enthusiasm and skepticism. The enthusiasm has stemmed from the potential these clinics have offered for meeting the acute and complex health needs of our nation's young people, particularly those in impoverished environments in which health care access has been limited. My own representative, Rep. Cardiss Collins has been instrumental in the implementation of these programs. Skepticism comes primarily from the focus of school based clinics on pregnancy prevention. This committee observed that while national rates of births by teenage parents have been declined from 1970 to 1982, pregnancy rates among teenagers have nearly doubled.

Unfortunately, the debate on the utility of school based health clinics has been drawn along partisan lines. Given these political considerations, it might be information to purse the question from a purely scientific perspective. All parties would seemingly agree that teenage health is a major national concern. Likewise, all would agree that pregnancy represents a major threat to the life long wellbeing of teenagers, particularly adolescent girls. The policy issue then becomes what is the best mechanism to address this problem. That is, how do we reduce the number of teenage pregnancies. From a scientific perspective, the controversy over the role of school based health clinics in pregnancy prevention, can be reduced into a clearly addressable question. Do school based clinic programs reduce the rate of pregnancy among the children and adolescents they serve?

And, if so, what are the characteristics of those programs that are the most effective and the least effective?

Regardless of political persuasion or prior belief about the efficacy of these clinics, it is unlikely that the validity of posing this scientific question is particularly controversial. However, answering this question through the use of existing empirical research, represents an important challenge fraught with the potential for controversy. Traditional reviews of the literature are often questioned based on selection of articles to be reviewed and different criteria used to evaluate one article than another. In order to review a literature in a fashion that cannot be criticized based on arbitrary decisions regarding articles, the selection of articles and criteria on which they are evaluated must be formally specified and reliably applied. This technique of literature review, first proposed by Light & Pillemer (1984), is called systematic analysis. I, along with a number of colleagues have used systematic analyses to study such issues as nursing home care and the effects of aggressive pornography on violence towards women.

In order to study the efficacy of school based clinics, we undertook a systematic analysis of the existing scientific literature. For the present analysis, a computerized Medline and PsychLit search from 1976 to 1990 identified 100 articles on school based clinics. Thirty-four (34%) were empirical studies, in that they reported at least one summary numeric result. Nearly two-thirds of the articles were non-empirical and included literature reviews, commentaries, and editorials.

The 34 empirical studies generally did not address the range of possible range of services proposed for school based clinics. Rather, 25 (76%) focused almost exclusively on pregnancy and contraception issues and services. Only five of these studies included any measures of other health concerns. Seven studies (21%) focused on prenatal or postnatal health services.

None of these studies investigated educational programs which emphasized abstinence as a form of pregnancy prevention, although several did study the effects of clinic operation on the onset and frequency of sexual behavior. This absence of abstinence research is compared to 21 studies focusing on contraception (primarily condoms and birth control bills) and six studies concentrating on abortion. One study investigated the role of adoption as an option to the resolution of unwanted pregnancy.

Eight studies were retrospective or prospective evaluations of the impact of clinic programs on sexual activity, contraception, pregnancy, and/or birth rates. On these four dependent variables the results across studies can be summarized as follows:

Sexual Activity. There is little evidence that clinics reduce or delay sexual activity. On the other hand, there appear to be no consistent evidence that clinics stimulate more sexual activity. On this dimension, the programs appear to be generally inert.

Contraception. There is fairly consistent evidence that clinics increase teenagers access to contraceptives. Clinics generally report fairly high utilization. There is substantially less evidence to show that contraception, provided by the clinics, is used more often (usually measured by asking whether contraception was used at last intercourse). Studies of knowledge about contraception increases, it does not become perfect.

Pregnancy. There is little consistent evidence that clinic programs effect pregnancy rates one way or the other. While some studies report modest declines, others report increases.

Birth Rates. There is fairly consistent evidence that school based health clinics do reduce birth rates. The mechanism for this effect, however, does not appear to be due to a reduction in pregnancy. Rather birth rates appeared to be reduce primarily through the use of abortion.

SUMMARY

Ideally, a well-functioning school based clinic should have a range of therapeutic services designed to meet the varying needs of school aged children. These might include, among other services, immunization, vision and hearing screening, and counseling services. The scientific evaluation literature on these clinics, however, has clearly focused on their role in pregnancy prevention. On this basic dimension, school based health clinics appear to fail to meet their mandate.

A good pregnancy prevention program should have the following outcomes:

1. A reduction in sexual activity and/or a reduction in the absolute number of unprotected sexual encounters.
2. As a direct effect of outcome 1, a reduction in the number of pregnancies.

It does not appear that school based health clinics achieve either of these two outcomes. Although admittedly selected for their impact, three quote from a recent study by Kirby, Waszak, & Ziegler (1991) dramatize the problem:

"In sum, simply providing contraceptives was not enough to significantly increase their use." (p 15)

"analysis of post data for the San Francisco clinic revealed that females (but not males) were significantly more likely to have sex than they had been before the clinic opened" (p 11)

"Clinic presence was not associated with lower rates of pregnancy at any sites, either during the previous 12 months or at any other time. In Dallas, the proportion of females who reported they had ever been pregnant was higher at the clinic school than at the comparison school." (p 14)

In discussing the findings, these authors were supportive of the clinic endeavors; however, their data, consistent with that of previous studies, portrays six school based clinic programs as failing to meet their goals of pregnancy prevention. The authors noted that those clinics with a larger educational program that emphasized responsibility in sexual relations and follow-up care appeared to be somewhat more effective than the others. This observation is consistent with a recently published study by Howard & McCabe (1990) reporting successful reductions in sexual activity through the use of an educational program that emphasized premarital abstinence.

Teenage pregnancy is one of the greatest risks in the "risky business of adolescence". When this committee decides how best to pursue a public policy to address this problem, I hope you will consider the findings of the scientific literature that suggest that school based health clinics may not be an effective means of helping our children.

John S. Lyons, Ph.D.

Associate Professor of Psychiatry, Psycholgy, & Medicine

References

Howard, M., & McCabe, J.P. (1990). Helping teenagers postpone sexual involvement. Family Planning Perspectives, 22: 21-26.

Kirby, D, Waszak, C., Ziegler, J. (1991). Six school-based clinics: Their reproductive health services and impact on sexual behavior. Family Planning Perspectives, 23, 6-16.

Light, RJ, & Pillemer, D.B. (1984). Summing Up: The Science of Reviewing. Harvard University Press, Cambridge, MA.

47-042 - 92 - 4

Chairwoman SCHROEDER. Thank you very much.

Now we will move along to our next witness. We really want to welcome this morning Ms. Bronwyn Mayden, and she is accompanied by Cathy Cardall.

The floor is yours, and thank you.

STATEMENT OF BRONWYN MAYDEN, EXECUTIVE DIRECTOR, MARYLAND GOVERNOR'S COUNCIL ON ADOLESCENT PREGNANCY; ACCOMPANIED BY CATHY CARDALL, PARENT OF A MEMBER OF THE HEALTH OPPORTUNITIES FOR TEENS ADVISORY BOARD, BALTIMORE, MD

Ms. MAYDEN. Thank you. Good morning, Madame Chairwoman and members of the committee. It is a pleasure for me to be here to testify for the Maryland Governor's Council on Adolescent Pregnancy and what we have been able to accomplish in the State of Maryland.

What I would like to do is just to give you some background on the Governor's Council. We were mandated several years ago by the General Assembly, and it is our goal to begin to decrease teen pregnancy in the State of Maryland, as well as to try to promote positive outcomes for pregnant teenagers, as well as for their families.

In addition to that, we look at public policy. I am the director for a public policy group, and what we have been doing is looking at the research, some of which you have heard reported today, in relationship to adolescent pregnancy to best chart which is the most effective way for the State of Maryland to pursue our goals.

And from looking at the research, we have come up with several strategies that I would like to talk with you about today.

The first strategy that we have been promoting in the State of Maryland is one of attempting to delay sexual initiation among teenagers. Basically this is an abstinence based program. It is for teenagers who are not sexually active, and we are trying to be very supportive of them.

Our research shows that we can most make impact on young people between the ages of nine to 14 years of age. So consequently, the materials that we have developed, which are posters, radio ads, TV ads, bus billboards, billboards all over the State of Maryland, really speak to that issue.

This is a program called Campaign for Our Children. The focus, each year we take a different focus, a different theme, and this year's theme happens to be male responsibility, and what I would like to do—I hope your eyes are not as bad as mine—but what I would like to do is to just show you some posters that we have developed around the issue of male responsibility.

The first poster says, "A baby costs $474 a month. How much do you have in your pocket? Babies are expensive," and we go on to talk about the state law, about how fathers are financially responsible for the children until the age of 18. If you do not help, the court will find you and make you pay child support even if you are not married. "So before you decide to have sex, see if you have a spare $100,000. Child support, you play, you pay."

The second one, "it is amazing how many guys disappear when one of these shows up". The same type of message at the bottom.

And the third, my favorite, is "What do you call a guy who makes a baby and flies the coop?" And we have a chicken. It is really a cock, but we call it a chicken. "A real man takes responsibility for his action. If a girl gets pregnant, he has to do the right thing. He doesn't cut and run," that type of thing. "Be a man. Be responsible."

These materials are in every public school in the State of Maryland, along with commercials, and radio, TV ads. This is a public-private partnership that our state put together, and we have raised $3.2 million for the use of all of this material.

The second strategy that we feel very, very strongly about because we know that most of the teens in our state are sexually active, is that we feel that we must begin to increase access to contraceptives to young people, and our Governor has been a forerunner in the State of Maryland in terms of providing additional funding for family planning clinics for teenagers.

We have a clinic in a mall, in a shopping area that has the highest teen pregnancy in the State of Maryland, along with the infant mortality rate. It is open in the evenings. It is open on weekends because from our research, what we have found is that clinics, whether they be school-based health clinics, are not accessible to teenagers, particularly in the summertime. They are not accessible to teenagers who are outside of school, who have unfortunately dropped out and have given up on the system.

So consequently, we have been putting a lot of our money and time in regard to providing contraceptive services for teens. Contraceptive services for teens, along with information, along with outreach so that they know where to come, along with services that we can provide for them on site.

We also know from some studies, and you have been hearing about some studies, that a correlation between the availability of family planning services and the probability of adolescent girls initiating sexual behavior, we have found that that is just not true, and there are numerous studies that have held constant many different factors that you begin to look at to see if that is true, and we have found that it is not true.

In addition, our state is a forerunner in the Three for Free Program. It is a condom distribution program that our state has had in operation since 1986. We provide condoms all over the state, anywhere that we can get in, bars, barber shops, beauty salons, restaurants, recreation centers. You name it; we provide condoms. We have provided almost four million condoms in 1990 alone at a cost of about $90,000.

Now, people wonder whether we are encouraging sexual behavior by providing condoms to young people, and I have to say to you we are not. What we are encouraging is to be responsible in terms of their sexual behavior.

This program was created from the demand of citizens that found that they wanted it. You ask me whether a program like this can work. Let me give you some data in terms of just Baltimore City.

In 1988, over one million condoms were given out at 134 locations in Baltimore City alone. During 1988, the occurrence rate of new cases of gonorrhea in Baltimore City dropped approximately

20 percent, and the rate of new cases of syphilis dropped 18 percent.

During the same time period on the East Coast, both of those diseases, you will find, had enormous increases in rates.

In our state the cost of a low birthweight baby, one, the lifetime cost, is around $400,000. The average Medicaid cost to support a person with AIDS from diagnosis to unfortunately death is around $22,000 in the State of Maryland.

I have to say to you that the mere $90,000 that the states puts into a condom distribution program, such as our Three for Free Program, we think, is very, very cost effective.

Finally, we have been working with parents around the issue of talking to their children about sex, and you have heard some comments from SIECUS, which I think we would like to really echo and say that we use quite a bit of their material in terms of getting parents to talk to kids about sex.

We have developed a program called PACT, which is Parents and Children Talking, because we feel also that parents are the educators of their children in regard to this issue, and we try to empower them by providing them with information and brochures and services in terms of this.

We had, during the month of October, about 150 events, all across the state for parents to get information in regards to sexuality for their kids, and actually we are going to do a pilot program in one of our counties that has the highest abortion rate to see if we can try to do a little bit more in terms of working with the local media down there.

And finally, the last thing that we fund are community organizations that want to work on the issue of adolescent pregnancy. My office is in Baltimore, and I do policy work. However, it has to be the community that decides to really stand up and address the issue of adolescent pregnancy in the manner that they feel best

So consequently, we provide money for community groups, and one of the community groups that we are giving money for is a school-linked clinic in relationship to adolescent health.

Now you have just heard some statistics in regards to school-based clinics and whether they are effective. I find it very interesting that perhaps some of the major research that has been done in relationship to school linked clinics was done at Johns Hopkins University with the Self-Clinic around 1984.

I hope that you are aware of this clinic. It is a clinic that has provided contraceptive services, and I think that that must be mentioned; that what we are finding from some of the research is that we are not providing a full range of services. Without a full range of services, we are not going to be successful.

What are the full range of services that we need? We are finding the kids that are coming into our school-based clinics need more information in terms of mental health services. If you look at the services that they come in to ask for, reproductive information, contraceptive services is very far down on the list. Usually it is young men that are coming in because they want to join basketball leagues, and they need sports physicals or physicals for jobs.

So consequently, these are the types of things that are going on in school-based clinics, and not that we are just handing out condoms or pushing pills down little girls' throats.

What we are seeing is that if we provide information, if we provide services, and if we provide contraceptive services, you will find that the teen pregnancy rates will go down.

In addition, in Baltimore, we were able to prove at our Self-Center that not only did the rates go down. The abortions went down, but not only that. We found that we had a probability of delaying sexual initiation by seven months for young women that we were able to pull into the clinics and to provide with information.

We know that these types of programs really do work, and what we need you to do is to provide us with funding to help us in terms of branching out and expanding the services. We have approximately ten school-based clinics in the State of Maryland right now.

With that I would like to thank you.

[Prepared statement of Bronwyn Mayden follows:]

PREPARED STATEMENT OF BRONWYN MAYDEN, EXECUTIVE DIRECTOR, MARYLAND GOVERNOR'S COUNCIL ON ADOLESCENT PREGNANCY, BALTIMORE, MD

Madame Chairwoman and members of the committee it is a pleasure for me to testify before the Select Committee on Children, Youth and Families on the efforts of Maryland Governor's Council on Adolescent Pregnancy to reduce unintended childbearing among adolescents.

The Council follows several strategies to reduce teen pregnancy. Different strategies because the Council realizes that adolescents are not a monolith group and that different strategies are needed to combat teen pregnancy.

The first strategy is to delay sexual initiation among youngsters. A media education program, Campaign For Our Children was developed that combines television and radio commercials, lesson plans, a video, buttons and t-shirts to bring the message to adolescents through schools, the community, and churches. Campaign For Our Children's theme for this year is male responsibility, and all the materials are developed around that topic. Using slogans like: "You Play , You Pay", "A baby costs $474 a month. How much do you have in your pocket? "and "What do you call a guy who makes a baby and flies the coop?" the Campaign utilizes media materials with a hands on program. Lesson plans that illustrate the cost of adolescent pregnancy, and its consequences are incorporated into the program. This highly successful public private partnership has raised approximately 3.2 million from state government and the business community.

The second strategy the Council uses to prevent adolescent pregnancy is expanding programs that provide access to contraception. Over 50% of 15-19 year old women and 80% of young men in the same age group are sexually active. It is important that this population have access to family planning services that provide a variety of health, education, and counseling services related to birth control including contraceptive services, pregnancy testing and counseling and information referral. In Maryland, Governor William Donald Schaefer has made a commitment to improving the accessibility of health services to young people and he has increased the budget for family planning services to teens by $2 million dollars annually. These funds have been used to open a teen clinic in a shopping mall, a clinic in a community center and outreach workers to inform teens of the services. All teen family planning clinics have changed their hours of operation so that they have evening and some have Saturday hours. The state has funded a number of school based health clinics that provide a variety of health services including contraceptives.

The Maryland Department of Health and Mental Hygiene leads the country in condom distribution with its Three for Free program. Condoms are distributed in quantities of 3 to 15 and instructional material on correct condom use are provided in non-medical settings, where young men congregate. Typical sites include pool halls, barber shops, recreation centers, college campuses, restaurants, and gas stations. In 1990, the Three for Free program with it s 454 sites gave away 3,098,879 condoms in Maryland. The program's cost of $90,000 is small if we are able to prevent a teen pregnancy or sexually transmitted diseases.

The third strategy that the Council uses is promoting information to parents to talk to their children about human sexuality. Parents should be the sexual educators of their children, however only 20% of parents talk to their children about sex. The Council through its Parents and Children Talking (PACT!) month encourages parents and children to talk about teenage sexual activity, adolescent pregnancy and contraception. PACT! talks, forums and workshops take place in more than 150 schools, health clinics, churches and recreations centers around the State of Maryland. Giant supermarkets and McDonalds restaurants display PACT! posters and brochures, "How to Talk to Your Kids about Sex". Maryland public libraries make books on the subject available.

The last strategy is empowering the community by providing funding for innovative projects that seek to prevent teen pregnancy. Funds are made available to organizations that want to develop comprehensive programs by linking existing services; fill in the gaps between existing services; and leverage private sector support for the proposed service. Currently we are funding eight projects including a school linked health clinic, mentoring program, after school program, and dollar a day program. The pregnancy rate for teens in all the programs is much lower than national averages or state averages.

Although the State of Maryland has done much to prevent adolescent pregnancy we need to do much more. Nationally, we need to make young people a priority. We must begin to change the political will and begin to:

- **Guarantee all adolescents access to health services regardless of ability to pay.** These services should be convenient, confidential, comprehensive and age appropriate. This will require the expansion of direct service, public health and school health services, and establishing adolescent health centers.

- **Schools must play a stronger role in improving adolescent health.** Schools can no longer accomplish their mission by ignoring the emotional and physical needs o f students. They need to provide information that teaches skills and information of accessing services. They should make arrangements for students to receive needed services, and increase their capacity to provide services.

- **Provide services where people are located.** Services need to be provided in the communities where adolescents and their families live. Providers need to be trained to work effectively with this population. Neighborhood outreach workers are needed to help adolescents and their families use health and other services to improve their life prospects.

- **Establish a federal Commission On Adolescent Pregnancy Prevention** that will fulfill the critical need for national leadership in mobilizing statewide efforts aimed at decreasing teen pregnancy. The Commission should:

  - ☐ Be comprised of cabinet secretaries, members of the Congress, the business community, academia, and local communities. It should be mandated to be a strong advocate in ensuring the development of a coordinated and comprehensive approach to the social, educational, economic, health, and problems of adolescent pregnancy.

- ❑ In cooperation with appropriate State and local agencies the Commission should foster plans to enhance coordination of all federally funded programs and services regarding adolescent pregnancy and parenthood in accordance with federal law.

- ❑ Promote the development of federal policies designed to enhance adolescent pregnancy prevention efforts and to improve services to at-risk, pregnant, and parenting adolescents.

- ❑ Monitor state-wide progress towards the goal of reducing adolescent pregnancy. Collect data and perform analysis of ongoing and new efforts aimed at reducing, preventing, and improving services to at-risk, pregnant, parenting adolescents.

- ❑ Establish a funding mechanism to distribute community incentive grants concerning adolescent pregnancy giving priority to innovative projects that:
  - ❑*Promote the establishment of a coordinated network of services for at-risk pregnant, and parenting adolescents;*
  - ❑*Demonstrate a high level of commitment to the project by making available funding, personnel, and facilities;*
  - ❑*Report to the President and the Congress on the level of expenditures and on the impact of programs and services regarding adolescent pregnancy and parenthood.*

Teen pregnancy is a complex phenomenon involving concepts of personal worth and identity; social norms and pressures; the allure of taking pleasure while avoiding responsibility; and economic deprivation. This complexity demands a comprehensive response aimed at achieving the goal of reducing teen pregnancy. This is an issue that demands the leadership, the long-term commitment, and the courage to expand or initiate many of the approaches you have heard about today. The urgency of the problem of teen pregnancy in human terms compels us to move forward quickly and boldly. Thank you.

Chairwoman SCHROEDER. Thank you very much. We really appreciate it.

Cathy, did you want to add anything?

Ms. CARDALL. Yes. I was asked to speak today from the perspective of a parent of a child who is involved in one of these outreach programs. So I would like to talk about that for just a minute.

I am the parent of six children, including three teenagers. So I clearly have a vested interest in exploring and being supportive of efforts aimed at helping adolescents stay safe.

When my daughter, Kirsten, was invited to serve on the Teen Advisory Board of the Health Opportunities for Teens Program, I encouraged her participation. I felt she would have something both to give and to gain. I knew she would be enthusiastic about giving input, and because we discussed these issues openly at home, I knew she would feel comfortable offering suggestions or presenting this information to other teenagers.

I also knew she would benefit by actively thinking about and discussing these topics with her peers and with the professional staff at the health center. I felt it would be a learning experience for her to see how other parents and kids deal with some of these issues.

I feel that I have been very lucky in establishing an open line of communication with my kids, and I have made this a priority. It seems that most parents do not have any problem talking to their kids when they are little. We tell them to look both ways when they cross the street and not to talk to strangers.

But too many stop the dialogue right at the point where our kids are most vulnerable and where even more serious dangers threaten them.

It is difficult to discuss adult things with our children, and by the time we see them as adults, they have already had to make a lot of adult decisions. In an ideal world, we could tell our teenagers to just say no, and they would. We could all openly and easily give them the information they need to stay safe, safe from sexually transmitted diseases, safe from drug and alcohol abuse, safe from AIDS. Unfortunately this does not always happen.

Not giving teenagers this information is like sending them unarmed into battle. Every time they leave the house, they are bombarded with pressures to make choices, and these must be informed sources.

It is clear that personal values and fear of pregnancy or disease do not stop some teenagers from having sex. So it becomes our responsibility to empower them, as Bronwyn was saying, with the information and support to make safe choices.

We need to have programs like the Health Opportunity for Teens or HOT, which are teen-friendly and create an open forum for discussion of all the areas which affect the teenager's decision-making process, things like self-esteem and stress and peer pressure.

These programs are also important because sometimes the pressures that the teenager feels stem from the home. Even in the best circumstances, this is a time when an adolescent search for self involves a rejection of his parents and their moral judgments. No matter where you look, you find good kids making bad choices.

A teenager needs a safe place to come to terms with his responsibility to himself, to his emotional and physical health. This becomes vitally and urgently important when he is considering behavior which can have a profound effect not only on the adolescent he is, but on the adult he is to become.

Chairwoman SCHROEDER. Thank you.

The chair wants to recognize the distinguished member who joined us in the audience, listening to all of you, from Baltimore. He must be very proud of this group. Congressman Mfume, thank you. We are very proud of them, too.

It is very rare that a member shows up to listen to testimony from your district. So that is very impressive. You have made an impression.

Dr. Hayton, we now yield to you, and we welcome you this morning, and we will look forward to hearing what you have to add.

STATEMENT OF BRADLEY P. HAYTON, PH.D., PUBLIC POLICY RESEARCH MANAGER, FOCUS ON THE FAMILY, POMONA, CA

Dr. HAYTON. I thank the Honorable Pat Schroeder for inviting me and the rest of the committee.

Essentially my talk is on the failure of condom-based sex education. Many schools administrators, as you know, have a great problem with teenage pregnancy, and with the best intentions they have distributed condoms or teach their students how to use condoms. They believe sincerely that such education will reduce teenage pregnancy, teenage illegitimacy and STDs, including AIDS.

Though the motives are good, the research just does not bear it out, and some sex education programs that promote the use of condoms increase teenage pregnancy rates, abortion rates, premarital sex, STDs and lower grades and academic aspirations.

Sex education programs that stress condom use tend to increase teenage pregnancy. Family planning agencies were established in the United States with an explicit goal of decreasing teenage pregnancy. Teaching adolescents to use contraceptives is their primary goal, but the effect really has just been the opposite.

The U.S. Senate Committee on Labor and Human Resources demonstrated a high correlation between federal programs and teenage pregnancy. Likewise, Olsen and Weed found that greater adolescent involvement in family planning programs was highly correlated with higher teenage pregnancies and higher teenage abortion rates.

Any net reduction in teenage births was due to the increased rates of abortion rather than the use of contraceptives. Five years ago this same committee, the U.S. Select Committee on Children, Youth, and Families, found that abortion, not contraceptives, was bringing about the reduction in teenage births, and the programs were not reducing the rates of teenage pregnancy and abortions.

Those states with the highest expenditures on family planning and with similar socio-demographic characteristics showed the largest increases of abortions and illegitimate births.

When comparing selective states to the national average, there was a high correlation between family planning funding and teenage pregnancy and abortion rates. Even studies by Planned Parenthood indicate a strong correlation between condom use and teenage pregnancy in their own programs.

What are some of the reasons? You know, why is this occurring? One is the failure rate of condoms. In the paper I have talked about a lot of the different statistics on the failure rate of condoms. Another reason is that the use of condoms increases teenage promiscuity, and there is much research to demonstrate that. And the third, which is mostly just common sense, although the research demonstrates that, too, is the impulsivity of teenagers. Even though they know when to use condoms, they do not use them.

So secondly, sex ed. programs that stress condom use increase abortion rates. Over and over a high correlation has been demonstrated between teenage abortions and these programs. One study by the CDC showed that 50 percent of the teenagers who got abortions had been using contraceptives at the time of conception. Pregnant teenage girls are far more likely to seek an abortion if they are unmarried than if they are married.

What are the effects of abortion? Of course, there are many physiological effects and psychological effects which have been studied many times, and I will not talk about all of the different effects abortion has.

Third, sex ed. programs that promote condoms encourage teenage promiscuity. In a survey of 400 randomly selected family physicians and psychiatrists, the majority agreed that the availability of contraceptives had led to an increased promiscuity among teenagers.

Planned Parenthood concluded, "Prior exposure to a sex education course is positively and significantly associated with the initiation of sexual activity at ages 15 and 16."

The National Research Council pointed out that the increased rate of sexual activity in teens, "is directly related to birth control information and provision to adolescents."

Dawson likewise concluded, "Prior contraceptive education increases the odds of starting intercourse at the age of 14 by a factor of 1.5." That is a 50 percent increase.

What are the effects of teenage pregnancy upon youth? Many. One is sexually active teenagers tend to drink alcohol and use marijuana more often and to smoke more, tend to have minor delinquency and school difficulty, and even an increased rate of suicide.

At the same time, early sexual experience is highly correlated with sexual promiscuity for the rest of life. The Redbook Report for Female Sexuality that interviewed 100,000 women found that if adolescents have sex by age 15, they are twice as promiscuous for the rest of their lives, and they are the least likely to rate their marriages or marital sex as good.

Number four. Sex ed. programs that stress condom use increase sexually transmitted diseases. Though as many as 75 percent of all the sexually active teens use some form of contraceptives, teens are increasingly contracting STDs.

The Department of Health and Human Services Task Force concluded that there is no clinical data to support the value that condoms prevent the spread of a range of diseases, including syphilis, herpes, hepatitis B or HIV/AIDS.

Dr. Nicholas Fiumara, Director of the Massachusetts Department of Public Health, wrote many comments, and I will just read a summary. He says, "In summary then, the effectiveness makes the condom useless as a prophylactic against gonorrhea, and even under ideal conditions against syphilis."

Though many STDs can be cured, of course, as we have mentioned many times today, there is no cure for HIV/AIDS. Condom education that increases sexual teen promiscuity coupled with the high failure rate of condoms makes teens more likely to contract the HIV virus.

Condoms are even less effective in stopping the spread of HIV than other STDs. In one study, 30 female prostitutes and 16 persons from a hospital staff each tested ten latex condoms in vaginal intercourse. Six people dropped out. The condom rupture occurred at least once for seven of the remaining 40 persons. Overall condom rupture rate was five percent.

The study concluded, "Truly safe sex with an HIV positive partner using condoms is a dangerous illusion."

Other studies, and I have summarized many of the studies in my report, came up with the same results.

In sum, the chances of contracting AIDS from an infected partner range from five to 17 percent. Once contracted, almost sure death is the final result. Other experts agree. Dr. Harold Jaffa, CDC's Chief of Epidemiology, writes, "You just can't tell people it's all right to do whatever you want so long as you wear a condom. It's just too dangerous a disease to say that."

Dr. Theresa Crenshaw, immediate past president of the American Association of Sex Educators, counselors and therapists wrote, "[I]f the wrong information is given, the effort will fail. It will cause"—and that was the stress that she made—"it will cause death rather than prevent it. . . . Saying that use of condoms is 'safe sex' is in fact playing Russian roulette. A lot of people will die in this dangerous game."

Of course, others concur. Right now, as you know, there are many liability problems starting to occur around the United States because of the ineffectiveness of condoms. The infection due to a faulty condom could be a cause of action.

Secondly, any facility which distributes or stores condoms could be liable since many condoms become defective because of storage practices and distribution practices.

Fifth, sex education programs that stress condom use and encourage premarital sex lowers grades and academic aspirations. There is not as much research on that because people do not do that. They want to look at effects in other ways, but there is some research to indicate that such is the case.

So here are the programs that do not work. What are some of the programs that work? This is much more difficult, as Dr. Lyons pointed out. They do not research those programs very often.

Many have found a high correlation between religious values and kids that do not engage in sex as often. They found a high correlation between two-parent families and kids that are sexually abstinent and do not have STDs. They found a high correlation between strong cultural norms and low illegitimacy rates. "Strong cultural norms and values proscribing early premarital sexual activity" is the primary reason for the relatively low illegitimacy rates among the Mexican–Americans, for instance.

Then, fourthly, they found high correlations in just the limited amount of research on the abstinence based sex ed. programs. However, I have to admit that people who do the research on the abstinence programs are the ones carrying out the abstinence programs. So they might be biased. It is not some journals like you talked about, Dr. Lyons.

In sum, then although the administrators have very good intentions and governments and the funding has good intentions to lower teenage pregnancy, to lower sexually transmitted diseases, including HIV virus, and to also even lower abortion rates, those things have increased even though the illegitimacy rates have gone down because of higher abortion rates.

Thank you very much.

[Prepared statement of Bradley P. Hayton Ph.D., follows:]

Prepared Statement of Bradley P. Hayton, Ph.D., Public Policy Research Manager, Focus on the Family, Pomona, CA

The Failures of Condom-Based Sex Education

Many times school administrators believe that they are best serving the interests of their students by distributing condoms, or teaching their students to use condoms. They believe that such education will reduce teenage pregnancy, teenage illegitimacy, and sexually transmitted diseases, including AIDS.

Though the motives are good, the belief is false. In fact, school programs that encourage the use of condoms do the very things that school administrators are trying to curtail. In order to help school administrators make their best informed opinion about programs that promote the use of condoms, this essay summarizes much of the research about the effectiveness of those programs, by giving succinct arguments against them.

In sum, sex education programs that promote the use of condoms increase teenage pregnancy rates, abortion rates, rates of premarital sex, sexually transmitted diseases, and lowers grades and academic aspirations.

<u>Sex education programs that stress condom use increase teenage pregnancy.</u>

Many have concurred that illegitimate births among teen mothers pose a grave risk to modern society. Willard Gaylin concludes, "The unattached, unsupported, and immature teenage mother is a knife at the throat of modern culture and a mortgage on the future vitality and hope of, especially, the black population in major cities where teenage illegitimacy is now the condition of a majority of births."[1] Consequently, schools have attempted to curtail illegitimate births by curbing teenage pregnancies.

Family planning agencies were established in the United States with the explicit goal of decreasing teenage pregnancies. Teaching adolescents to use contraceptives is their primary goal. The effect, however, has been just the opposite.

The U.S. Senate Committee on Labor and Human Resources demonstrated a high correlation between federal programs and teenage pregnancy.[2] Likewise, Olsen and Weed found that greater adolescent involvement in family planning programs was correlated significantly with higher teenage pregnancies and higher teenage abortion rates. Any net reduction of teenage births was due to increased rates of abortion, rather than the use of contraceptives.[3]

The same is true for state programs. The U.S. Select Committee on Children, Youth, and Families found that abortion, not contraceptives, was bringing about the reduction in teen births.[4] And the programs were not reducing the rates of teenage pregnancy and abortions. Those states with the highest expenditures on family planning and with similar socio-demographic characteristics showed the largest increases in abortions and illegitimate births.[5] When comparing selective states to the national average, there is a high correlation between family planning funding and teenage pregnancy and abortion rates.[6]

Though the rate of births plus the rate of abortions had declined between 1957 and 1971, there began a step-by-step increase in adolescent pregnancy with new federally funded sex programs.[7] By 1982, almost 45 percent of all pregnancies of teenagers were being aborted.[8] "Not only did teenage pregnancy increase when government intervened to control it, but it was subsequently discovered that teenage pregnancy decreased when visits to the government-funded family-planning clinics declined," comments Jacqueline Kasun from Humbolt State University.[9]

Even studies by Planned Parenthood indicate a strong correlation between condom use and teenage pregnancy. They found, between 1976 and 1979, premaritally sexually active women aged 15-19 who always used contraceptives had 19.2 percent increased pregnancies. During the same period, the pregnancy rate among women who had always used contraceptives rose 36.4 percent.[10]

In sum, population researcher, Phillips Cutright, arrives at the conclusion, "We find no evidence that the programs reduced white illegitimacy, because areas with weak programs or no programs at all experience smaller increases or larger declines [in pregnancy] than are found in areas with strong contraceptive programs."[11] Research throughout the country continually confirms this belief.[12]

There are many reasons for a high correlation between condom use and increased teenage pregnancy. First, several have documented that the failure rate of condoms used by teenage girls to prevent pregnancy is 18.4%.[13] Condoms are notorious for leakage. According to the Department of Health and Human Services, "One of every five batches of condoms tested in a government inspection program over the last four months failed to meet minimum standards for leaks."[14] FDA agents reject one lot in ten of domestic condoms, and one in five of imported condoms.[15] Present FDA standards for lots acceptable for public sale allow up to four condoms per thousand to leak water.[16]

Zelnik and Kantner write in Planned Parenthood's journal, "Even among teens who use oral contraceptives regularly and follow the ideal pattern prescribed by Planned Parenthood, the pregnancy rate is 5.8 percent."[17] Using Planned Parenthood's statistics, Ruff has computed that an adolescent who uses condoms has an 87 percent likelihood of an unwanted pregnancy while she is in school.[18] Mishell found that among sexually active women under age twenty-five, up to one-third who use only condoms for contraception will be pregnant after one year.[19] Though condoms have an overall 10 percent failure rate when used for contraception,[20] it is almost twice as high for young people.[21]

Second, several studies have documented that the use of condoms increases teenage promiscuity.[22] And third, teenagers typically engage in sexual activities upon impulse, believe that condoms curtail sexual enjoyment, and do not use condoms properly.

Sex education programs that stress condom use increase abortion rates.

As noted above, sex ed programs that promote the use of condoms are highly correlated with teenage abortions. One study by the Centers for Disease Control (CDC) showed that 50 percent of teenagers who got abortions had been using contraceptives at the time of conception.[23] Pregnant teenage girls are far more likely to seek an abortion if they are unmarried than if they are married.[24]

There is a large body of statistical data and medical literature that demonstrates the lasting physical and psychological effects of abortion. These effects include the perforation of the uterus, laceration of the cervix, the injury to the bowel and bladder, hemorrhage, severe infection, cardiac arrest, convulsions, endotoxic shock, pulmonary embolism, thrombophlebitis, and sometimes death.[25] A plethora of studies have demonstrated that the proportion of babies delivered prematurely varied between 40 percent higher to almost three times as high among mothers who had previous abortions, compared to those who had not.[26] Premature birth is highly correlated with mental retardation and other health problems in children.[27] Harlap and Davies also found that prior abortions were also associated with high neonatal deaths and malformations in children subsequently born.[28] Last, several studies have indicated that women who have abortion have higher rates of infertility.[29]

Psychological consequences of abortion have been termed "post-abortion syndrome" by the psychiatric community. About 90 percent of women who have abortions experience moderate to severe emotional and psychiatric stress following an abortion. Reardon comments, "Up to 10 percent require psychiatric hospitalization or other professional treatment. One to two percent (15,000 to 30,000 women per year) suffer such severe trauma as to render them unable to work. In addition, aborted women face a suicide risk nine times greater than that of non-aborted women."[30]

These symptoms include: anxiety,[31] depression, guilt,[32] regret, anger, embarrassment, fear of disapproval, shame, insomnia, and remorse.[33] If not actually abandoned, many women _feel_ abandoned.[34] Many women feel sexual coldness or become frigid for periods of time.[35] Some react by becoming more promiscuous.[36] Many become more suicidal.[37]

Of course, these effects of abortion do not take into account the effects on the child of increased illegitimate teenage pregnancy. Pickering concludes that "the marital status of the mother was significantly associated with the risk of birth weight below 2,500 g [5.5 pounds] and 2,000 g [4.4 pounds]." Among women bearing a first child, the risk of low birth weight was 28 percent higher for unmarried mothers than for married mothers, and 63 percent higher for a second or subsequent child.[38]

Sex Ed Programs that promote condoms encourage teenage promiscuity.

Planned Parenthood has continually maintained "universal reproductive freedom" as their goal. As early as 1963, then-president Alan Guttmacher acknowledged that contraceptive information for teens would increase sexual promiscuity.[39]

Medical doctors who helped invent the pill have concurred. In 1977, Dr. Robert Kistner of Harvard Medical School said, "About 10 years ago I declared that the pill would not lead to promiscuity. Well, I was wrong."[40] In 1981, Dr. Min Chueh Chang commented, "I personally feel the pill has rather spoiled young people. . . . It's made them more permissive."[41]

In a survey of 400 randomly selected family physicians and psychiatrists, the majority agreed that the availability of contraceptives has led to increased promiscuity among teenagers.[42] Planned Parenthood concluded: "...[P]rior exposure to a sex education course is positively and significantly associated with the initiation of sexual activity at ages 15 and 16."[43] The National Research Council pointed out that the increased rate of sexual activity in teens "is directly related to birth control information and provision to adolescents."[44]

Dawson concluded that "Prior contraceptive education increases the odds of starting intercourse [at the age of 14] by a factor of 1.5," a 50 percent increase.[45]

Other researchers have confirmed these reports that contraceptive education is highly correlated with increased sexual activity.[46]

Teen-age sex, especially at 15-years-old or earlier, is especially dangerous to physical and psychological health. Several researchers have found high correlations between early sexual experience and alcohol and marijuana use.[47] Early sexual experience has also been linked with cigarette use,[48] minor delinquency, and school difficulty.[49] Nonvirginal girls are also over 6 times more likely to report having attempted suicide, are at slightly greater risk for reporting feeling lonely, feeling upset, and having difficulty sleeping,[50] as well as experience lower self-esteem.[51]

At the same time, early sexual experience is highly correlated with sexual promiscuity throughout the rest of life. The Redbook Report for Female Sexuality found that women who had sex by age fifteen are twice as promiscuous for the rest of their lives as women who didn't.[52] Even though later married these women were more likely to use marijuana while having sex, masturbate frequently, be turned on by pornography, and almost three times more likely to have a homosexual encounter.[53] They were also the least likely to rate their marriages or marital sex as good.

Sex ed programs that stress condom use increase sexually-transmitted diseases.

Though as many as seventy-five percent of all sexually active teens use some form of contraceptives,[54] teens are increasingly contracting venereal diseases. The annual in-use failure rate for condoms is over eighteen percent.[55]

Sexually active single teens are more likely than married women to be infected with an entire host of STDs, including M. hominis, G. vaginalis, yeasts, U. urealyticum, and T. vaginalis.[56] Likewise, teen mothers then carry infants suffering from pneumonia and other illnesses.[57]

A Department of Health and Human Services task force concluded that there are no clinical data to support the value that condoms prevent the spread of a range of diseases, including syphilis, herpes, hepatitis-B, and HIV.[58] Dr. Nicholas Fiumara, director of the Massachusetts Department of Public Health, wrote:

> The current epidemic of gonorrhea in the United States and in Massachusetts has prompted many physicians to ask us about the effectiveness of the condom as a prophylactic against this disease. The answer to this question is theoretically yes, but the effectiveness of the condom is such as to make it completely useless as a prophylactic.
>
> The condom is effective against gonorrhea provided there is no preliminary sex play, the condom is intact before use, the condom is put on correctly and the condom is taken off correctly. However, the male population has never been able to fulfill the very first requisite.
>
> Even if all these conditions are fulfilled, a condom incompletely protects against syphilis because it protects only the part it covers ... It does not cover ... the areas that are bathed with the secretion of the female during the sex act.
>
> In summary, then, its effectiveness makes the condom useless as a prophylactic against gonorrhea, and even under ideal conditions against syphilis.[59]

Though many STDs can be cured, there is no cure for HIV/AIDS. Condom education that increases teen promiscuity, coupled with the high failure rate of condoms, makes teens more likely to contract the deadly HIV virus. Condoms are even less effective in stopping the spread of HIV. In one study, thirty female prostitutes and sixteen persons from a hospital staff each tested ten latex condoms in vaginal intercourse. Six people dropped out, and condom rupture occurred at least once for seven of the remaining forty persons. Overall condom rupture rate was 5 percent. The study concluded, "Truly safe sex with an HIV-positive partner using condoms is a dangerous illusion."[60]

Other studies have confirmed these results. In married couples in which one partner was HIV-infected and condoms were used, 10 percent of the healthy became infected within two years.[61] Though condom usage was shown to decrease HIV acquisition among prostitutes and monogamous couples, the same study confirmed HIV is also spread to the uninfected.[62] In fact, Fischl and her colleagues found that couples who exclusively used condoms showed a 17 percent seroconversion rate over a 12-18 month period. Using condoms for HIV protection is such a poor practice that another study, conducted by the federal government in the Los Angeles area, was ultimately withdrawn in August 1988 because participants were placed at too great a risk of contracting the virus.[63]

In sum, the chances of contracting AIDS from an infected partner range from 5-17 percent.[64] Once contracted, almost sure death is the final result. The chances of contracting other STDs are about the same. Condom "safe sex" is a myth.

Experts agree. Dr. Harold Jaffe, CDC's chief of epidemiology, writes, "You just can't tell people it's all right to do whatever you want so long as you wear a condom. It's just too dangerous a disease to say that."[65] Dr. Theresa Crenshaw, immediate past president of the American Association of Sex Educators, Counselors and Therapists, and member of the Presidential AIDS commission, says, "[I]f the wrong information is given, the effort will fail. It will <u>cause</u> death rather than prevent it.... Saying that use of condoms is 'safe sex' is in fact playing Russian roulette. A lot of people will die in this dangerous game."[66]

Others concur. Dr. Bruce Voeller, president of the Mariposa Research Foundation, which specializes in the prevention of sexually transmitted diseases, writes, "The safe sex message just isn't true. You're still playing a king of Russian roulette."[67] Dr. Malcolm Potts, one of the inventors of condoms lubricated with spermicides, and president of Family Health International: "We cannot tell people how much protection condoms give."[68] Telling a person who engages in high-risk behavior to use a condom "is like telling someone who is driving drunk to use a seat belt."[69] Even Mayor Ed Koch of New York City commented, "It is a misnomer, a fraud, to try to convey to people that if they use condoms they're absolutely safe from contracting AIDS. Just as it is a fraud to say if you use condoms, there's no danger of pregnancy."[70]

As a result, many are starting to be concerned about the possible product liabilities as a result of the ineffectiveness of condoms. Since even with proper use infection may occur, infection due to a faulty condom could be a cause of action. And since the storage of condoms often times lowers their effectiveness, the facility which distributes and stores condoms could be liable.[71]

<u>Sex ed programs that stress condom use and encourage premarital sex lowers grades and academic aspirations.</u>

At least for white males, grades take a huge drop when teens begin engaging in premarital sex. Among white females, sexual intercourse appears to depress the academic aspirations, reducing the personal emphasis on school work and the desire to go to college. These, in turn, may considerably alter these teens' later life.[72]

In sum, these are key arguments against selling condoms in high school vending machines. Such a policy works against many of the government intentions in curtailing teen pregnancy, teen abortion, teen promiscuity, and teen sexually transmitted diseases, as well as decreases academic aspirations and achievement.

If the public school system wishes to achieve these ends with teenagers, other policies make much more sense. Many studies have demonstrated decreased teen pregnancy, abortion, and promiscuity have these correlates.

1. Religion. Many studies have shown that more religious adolescents engage in less sexual behavior with their peers.[73] Several studies have demonstrated that the "erosion of traditional values related to marriage and family and sexual behavior" is one of the primary causes of "date rape."[74]

2. Two-parent families. Both males and females raised in single parent homes are a great deal more likely to become unwed teen mothers or fathers.[75] Teenage girls also suffer the humiliation of involuntary intercourse least when they live with both parents.[76] Knight and Prentky found that a sizeable majority of rapists come from single-parent homes.[77]

Adolescents reared in single-parent households engage in sexual intercourse earlier and more often than those reared in intact families.[78] Adolescent girls who live with both parents are also less likely to bear a child in their early teens than adolescent girls who only live with their mothers.[79] Likewise, teenage children of traditional mothers who stay home engage in sexual activity much less often than peers raised by career women.[80] Even teens from large families are less likely to engage in premarital sex than teens from small families.[81] Daughters of divorced parents are much more likely to plan for nonmarital cohabitation that are the daughters of intact homes.[82]

3. Strong cultural norms. Many researchers have found that "strong cultural norms and values proscribing early premarital sexual activity" is the primary reason for the relatively low illegitimacy rates among, for example Mexican Americans, as compared to Blacks.[83] Young Hispanic women from intact families who regularly attend church usually refrain from sexual activity before marriage.[84] Adolescent Hispanic women who have recently immigrated from Mexico are even more likely to remain abstinent until marriage.[85] In contrast, single-parent black families tend to raise unwed teen mothers.[86] Rowe and St. John contend that the cause by a "culture of premarital childbearing" where daughters are less likely to perceive "moral and social disapproval for being sexually active."

4. Abstinence-based sex ed programs. In contrast to the typical sex ed classes or school-based clinics that promote condoms, abstinence-based sex ed programs are showing great success in curtailing teen pregnancy and teen promiscuity. The AANCHOR project was tested for five years in thirteen school districts in Utah, California, New Mexico, and Arizona, and found correlations with 1) higher family strengths (loyalty, emotional support, cohesion), 2) more frequent discussions with parents about sexual values and beliefs, and 3) more abstinent attitudes regarding premarital sexual involvement.[87]

The Me, My World, My Future program, which is used by over 2,500 schools, was tested at four junior high schools during two months in 1988, and found correlations with 1) student awareness of the benefits of abstinence, 2) more likelihood of abstinence before marriage, 3) increased awareness of the negative consequences of teenage sexual behavior, and 4) a greater belief that premarital sexuality was against their values.[88] Sex Respect, adopted in over 1,000 school districts across the United States, in a study with 1,841 participants found high correlations with 1) abstinence attitudes, 2) a greater sense of sexual control by teens, and 3) a greater awareness of the benefits of abstinence.[89]

Sexuality, Commitment, and Family, used by San Marcos Junior High, decreased the pregnancies from 147 to 20 among their students, after only two years of implementation.[90] Other programs have demonstrated similar results.[91]

Conclusion

Selling condoms in vending machines in high school bathrooms will not curtail teenage pregnany. Study after study has demonstrated that condom education and condom distribution increases teen pregnancies, teen abortions, teen promiscuity, and teen sexually transmitted diseases.

If the public school system wishes to effectively deal with these serious problems of teenagers, then administrators must implement policies that will support the traditional family and teach traditional values, such as abstinence before marriage.

Endnotes

1. Willard Gaylin, Adam and Eve and Pinocchio: On Being and Becoming Human (New York: Viking, 1990), pp. 245-250.

2. Testimony before the U.S. Senate Committee on Labor and Human Resources, March 31, 1981, as cited in Joseph R. Peden and Fred R. Glahe, eds., The American Family and the State (San Francisco, CA: Pacific Research Institute for Public Policy, 1986), p. 355.

3. Joseph A. Olsen, & Stan Weed, "Effects of Family-Planning Programs for Teenagers on Adolescent Birth and Pregnancy Rates" and "Effects of Family-Planning Programs on Teenage Pregnancy--Replication and Extension," Family Perspective, Fall 1986, pp. 154-195; Wall Street Journal, October 14, 1986.

4. Report of the U.S. House Select Committee on Children, Youth, and Families, Teen Pregnancy: What Is Being Done? A State-By-State Look (Washington, D.C.: Government Printing Office, 1986), p. 20. Updated data from "Trends: Adolescent Pregnancy, Abortion, and Childbearing," Family Life Information Exchange (Rockville, MD, May 1987), pp. 1-4.

5. Testimony cited in Peden and Glahe, eds., The American Family, p. 356; Jacqueline R. Kasun, Teenage Pregnancy: What Comparisons among States and Counties Show (Stafford, VA: American Life League, 1986).

6. "In fifteen states with similar social-demographic characteristics and rates of teenage pregnancy in 1970, those with the highest expenditures on family planning showed the largest increases in abortions and illegitimate births among teenagers between 1970 and 1979." Jacqueline R. Kasun, The War Against Population (San Francisco, CA: Ignatius, 1988), as cited from Susan Roylance, Testimony before the U.S. Senate Committee on Labor and Human Resources, March 31, 1981.

7. Jacqueline R. Kasun, Testimony before the U.S. Senate Committee on Labor and Human Resources, March 31, 1981.

8. Jacqueline R. Kasun, The War Against Population (San Francisco, CA: Ignatius, 1988), pp. 143-144.

9. "In 1980 the state of Utah passed a law requiring parental consent for contraceptives given to minors. In the following year there was a decline in clinic attendance by teenagers, and the pregnancy rate--which had been increasing among girls of 15-17--declined for the age-group, as did abortion and birth rates." Kasun, The War Against Population, p. 144, citing Press release by United Families of America, March 8, 1983, quoting figures from Utah Department of Health.

10. Melvin Zelnik, & John F. Kantner, "Sexual Activity, Contraceptive Use, and Pregnancy Among Metropolitan-Area Teens: 1971-1979," Family Planning Perspectives, Vol. 12, 1980, cited in Josh McDowell, The Myths of Sex Education (San Bernardino, CA: Here's Life, 1990), p. 125.

11. Phillips Cutright, "Illegitimacy in the United States: 1920-1968," in Robert Parke, Jr., and Charles F. Westoff, Research Reports, U.S. Commission of Population Growth and the American Future, Vol. 1 (Washington, DC: Government Printing Office), p. 121.

12. Josh McDowell, The Myths of Sex Education (San Bernardino, CA: Here's Life, 1990) has obtained these quotes from leading authorities:

Richard Weatherly, Family Planning Perspectives (PPFA): "Comprehensive programs . . . are not the magic bullet that will solve the problems associated with unintended teenage pregnancy and parenthood. Nor should they be expected to do so." Richard Weatherly, et al., "Comprehensive Programs for Pregnant Teenagers and Teenage parents: How Successful Have They Been?," Family Planning Perspectives, Vol 18 (2), March/April 1986, p. 77.

Deborah Ann Dawson: "Prior contraceptive education increases the odds of starting intercourse at [the age of] 14 . . . . by 50 percent." "The Effects of Sex Education on Adolescent Behavior," Family Planning Perspectives, Vol. 18 (4), July/August 1986, pp. 168-9.

Senate subcommittee report: "With more than 5,000 'family planning clinics' operating in the United States, many of them with the help of federal funds, and sex education courses in many public schools, it is clear that contraceptive information alone is not the solution to the unwanted consequences of sexual activity." Michael J. McManus, ed., Final Report of the Attorney General's Commission on Pornography (New York: Rutledge Hill Press, 1986.

Congressional budget office report: "Since Title X federal funding for family planning programs began in 1971, the number of teenage girls in subsidized birth control programs increased 397 percent; who used contraceptives but became pregnant increased 266 percent; who had abortions increased 107 percent; who contracted an STD increased 93 percent." Action Line X, May 12, 1986, p. 4.

Dr. James W. Stout, Children's Hospital of Seattle: "Five studies conducted from 1980 to 1987 examined the effect of classroom sex education programs at the junior and senior high school level on teenagers from a variety of geographical areas and racial and socioeconomic groups. The researchers said: 'The programs had no discernible impact on pregnancy rates, a negligible effect on using birth control methods and insignificant influence on teenagers' decisions about when to engage the first time in sexual intercourse.'" James Stout, & Frederick P. Rivara, "Schools and Sex-Education: Does It Work?," Pediatrics, Vol 83 (3), March 1989.

Drs. James Stout and Federick P. Rivara in the medical journal Pediatrics: "Our findings indicate that the expectations of altered adolescent sexual activity, contraceptive behavior and pregnancy are unlikely to be fulfilled by these [school-based sex education] programs, and we suggest that the effort to fight for sex education on these terms is not justified unless an effect is shown in further studies. To place the burden of counteracting the prevailing forces in our society toward premarital sex on our schools alone is both naive and inappropriate." Ibid, pp. 375-379.

Former Secretary of Education William Bennett: "There is no evidence that making contraceptive methods more available is the surest strategy for preventing pregnancy -- to say nothing of preventing sexual activity. . . . Seventy percent of all high school seniors have taken sex eduction courses in 1985, up from 60 percent in 1976. Yet when we look at what is happening in the sexual lives of American students, we can only conclude that it is doubtful that much sex education is doing any good at all." William J. Bennett, "Our Children," Address to the National School Board of Education, January 22, 1987.

Dr. Larry Cuban, professor of education, Stanford University: "Decade after decade . . . statistics have demonstrated the ineffectiveness of such courses in reducing sexual activity [and] teenage pregnancy. In the arsenal of weapons to combat teenage pregnancy, school-based programs are but a bent arrow. However, bent arrows do offer the illusion of action." Ibid.

Hansen, Myers and Gisburg report in the Journal of Marriage and Family that their "findings suggest that knowledge as measured by birth control knowledge and sex education courses is not successful in reducing the change of out-of-wedlock childbearing. . . . These findings have important implications for programs and policies addressing teenage pregnancy and childbearing. Although sex education is often promoted as a way to reduce the incidence of early pregnancy, our results suggest that simply requiring more students to take more sex education as it is currently provided is not the answer." Journal of Marriage and Family, May 1987, pp. 241-56.

Dr. Deborah Ann Dawson, in Planned Parenthood's publication: "The NSFG [National Survey of Family Growth] data reveal no significant relationship between exposure to sex education and the risk of premarital pregnancy among sexually active teenagers. . . . The final result to emerge from the analysis is that neither pregnancy education nor contraceptive education exerts any significant effect on the risk of premarital pregnancy among sexually active teenagers -- a finding that calls into question the argument that formal sex education is an effective tool for reducing adolescent pregnancy." "The Effects of Sex Education on Adolescent Behavior," Family Planning Perspectives, Vol. 18 (4), July/August 1986, pp. 168-9.

13. Mark D. Hayward, & Jonichi Yogi, "Contraceptive Failure Rate in the United States: Estimates From the 1982 National Survey of Family Growth," Family Planning Perspectives, Vol. 18 (5), September/October 1986, p. 204; Melvin Zelnik, Michael A.K. Koenig, & Kim Young, "Sources of Prescriptive Contraceptives and Subsequent Pregnancy Among Young Women," Family Planning Perspectives, January/February 1984; "Update on Condoms -- Products, Production, Promotion," Population Reports, September/October, 1982, pp. H121-122.

14. Asta Kenney, "School-Based Clinics: A National Conference," Family Planning Perspectives, vol. 18 (1), January/February 1986, pp. 6, 28.

15. Consumer Reports, March, 1989, as cited in Josh McDowell, The Myths of Sex Education (San Bernardino, CA: Here's Life, 1990), p. 61; cf. "Condoms," Consumer Reports, October 1979, pp. 586-589, which are discussed by Voeller and Potts in British Medical Journal, October 26, 1986, p. 1196.

16. The acceptable quality level is 0.4%, or four leaky condoms per thousand. "The industry standard requires, roughly, that no more than four condoms out of 1,000 leak. The condoms are tested by pouring 10 ounces of water in each and looking for leakage." HHS News, June 19, 1987. Cf. also FDA, Compliance Policy Guidelines, chapter 24, guide 7124.21, April 10, 1987, p. 1: "The sampling inspection plan used by the FDA also emphasizes adequate protection against FDA rejecting lots where the percent defective is less that [sic] or equal to 0.4%."

17. Melvin, Zelnik, & John F. Kantner, "Contraceptive Patterns and Premarital Pregnancy Among Women Ages 15-19 in 1976," Family Planning Perspectives, Vol. 10 (3), May/June 1978, p. 138.

18. Robert Ruff, Aborting Planned Parenthood (Houston, TX: New Vision, 1988), pp. 66f.

19. D.R. Mishell, "Contraception," The New England Journal of Medicine, Vol. 320, 1989, pp. 777-787.

20. "Update on Condoms--Products, Protection, Promotion," Population Reports, September-October 1982, pp. H-121-H122.

21. William Grady, Mark Hayward, Junichi Yagi, "Contraceptive Failure in the United States: Estimates from the 1982 National Survey of Family Growth," Family Planning Perspectives, Vol. 18

(5), September/October 1986, pp. 203, 204, 207. This is also true internationally. In Indonesia, couples where wives were 15-24 years old had a 38 percent pregnancy rate, compared with 13 percent where wives were 25-35 years old (Grady, p. 207). A study of five Latin American countries found that the pregnancy rate was 17 percent for women under age 30 compared with 7 percent for women age 30 or above ("Update on Condoms--Products, Protection, Promotion," Population Reports, September-October 1982, pp. H-125).

22. New York Times, June 12, 1981, A16; P.A. Reichelt, "Changes in Sexual Behavior Among Unmarried Teenage Women Utilizing Oral Contraception," Journal of Population, Vol. 1, 1987, p. 57; A. Peitropino, "Survey on Contraception Analysis," Medical Aspects of Human Sexuality, May 1987, p. 147; S. DuBose Ravenal, "American Teens and Birth Control," North Carolina Medical Journal, Vol. 48, November 1987, p. 606; Jacqueline R. Kasun, "Sex Education: The Hidden Agenda," The World & I, Vol. 4 (9), September 1989, p. 495.

23. Frances Frech, "Update on Teen Pregnancies," Heartbeat Quarterly, Summer 1980.

24. Theodore Joyce, "The Social and Economic Correlates of Pregnancy Resolution Among Adolescents in New York City, by Race and Ethnicity: A Multivariate Analysis," American Journal of Public Health, Vol. 78, June 1988, pp. 626-630.

25. For a summary of the physiological and psychological effects, cf. David C. Reardon, Aborted Women: Silent No More (Westchester, IL: Crossway, 1987); also cf. Christopher Tietze, Induced Abortion: 1979, 3rd ed. (New York: The Population Council, 1979), pp. 79-81.

26. Leslie Iffy, et al., "Perinatal Statistics: The Effect Internationally of Liberalized Abortion," in Thomas W. Hilgers, et al., New Perspectives on Human Abortion (Frederick, ML: University Publications of America, 1981), pp. 92-127; John A. Richardson, & Geoffrey Dixon, "Effects of Legal Termination on Subsequent Pregnancy," British Medical Journal, Vol. 1, 1976, pp. 1303-1304; Hungarian Central Statistical Office, "The Effect of the Number of Abortions on Premature Births and Perinatal Mortality in Hungary," Budapest, 1972; Marriage and Family Newsletter, Vol. 4 (2-4), February, March, April, 1973; S. Harlap and A.M. Davies, "Late Sequelae of Induced Abortion: Complications and Outcome of Pregnancy and Labor," American Journal of Epidemiology, Vol. 102 (3), September 1975, pp. 217-224; Vito M. Logrillo, et al., Effect of Induced Abortion on Subsequent Reproductive Function, Final Report, New York State Department of Health, Office of Biostatistics, April 18, 1980, Contract no. N01-HD-6-2802, National Institute of Child Health and Human Development.

27. Dionne J. Jones, & Stanley F. Battle, eds., Teenage Pregnancy (New Brunswick, NJ: Transaction, 1990), p. 6; also John M. Taborn, "Adolescent Pregnancy: A Medical Concern," pp. 91-100 in Teenage

Pregnancy.

28. Ann Aschengrau Levin, et al., "Association of Induced Abortion with Subsequent Pregnancy Loss," Journal of the American Medical Association, Vol. 243 (24), June 27, 1980, pp. 2495-2499; for a review of the literature see, Karl E. Bauman, & Ann E. Anderson, "Legal Abortions and Trends in Fetal and Infant Mortality Rates in the United States," American Journal of Obstetrics and Gynecology, Vol. 136 (2), January 15, 1980, pp. 194-202.

29. Several times as high a proportion of women who have had an abortion are being treated for infertility, cf. D. Trichopoulos, et al., "Induced Abortion and Secondary Infertility," British Journal of Obstetrics and Gynecology, Vol. 83, August 1976, pp. 645-650; a New York study found that women who had aborted had 37 percent fewer pregnancies and less than half as many live births in the six following years than women who had not, cf. Vito M. Logrillo, et al., Effect of Induced Abortion on Subsequent Reproductive Function, Final Report, New York State Department of Health, Office of Biostatistics, April 18, 1980, Contract no. N01-HD-6-2802, National Institute of Child Health and Human Development.

30. David C. Reardon, Aborted Women, p. xxv.

31. Ann Saltenberger, Every Woman Has a Right to Know the Dangers of Legal Abortion (Glassboro, NJ: Air-Plus Enterprises, 1982), citing Kent, et al., pp. 136, 138, 140. Anxiety was reported by 43.1 percent surveyed.

32. Philip G. Ney, "Infant Abortion and Child Abuse: Cause and Effect," The Psychological Aspects of Abortion (Washington, DC: University Publications of America, 1979), p. 29. Severe guilt is found in 2 to 23 percent, depending upon the type of study, according to E.C. Moore-Caver, "The International Inventory on Information on Induced Abortion," International Institute for the Study of Human Reproduction, Columbia University, 1974. Also Ann Saltenberger above found depression with more than a moderate strength reported by 31.9 percent surveyed, 26.4 percent felt guilt, and 18.1 percent felt no relief or just a bit. Another study cited by Saltenberger found that 23 percent suffered 'severe guilt,' and an additional 25 percent experienced 'mild guilt' (p. 140). Various surveys in Japan demonstrate the same phenomenon there. Surveys have found that 73.1 percent of Japanese women report "anguish" about their abortion, 59 percent felt that abortion is something "very bad," 16 percent felt it was considerably bad, 17 percent felt it was somewhat bad, while only 8 percent thought it could not be considered bad (cf. John Willke, & Barbara Willke, Handbook on Abortion (Cincinnati: Hayes Publishing Co., 1979), p. 51, and; James T. Burtchaell, Rachel Weeping (New York: Harper & Row, 1984), pp. 104-105.

33. Ann Saltenberger, Every Woman Has a Right to Know the Dangers of Legal Abortion (Glassboro, NJ: Air-Plus Enterprises, 1982), pp. 138-146.

34. Linda Bird Francke, Ambivalence of Abortion (New York: Random House, 1978), pp. 47-48; Monte Harris Liebman, & Jolie Siebold Zimmer, "Psychological Sequelae of Abortion," in David Mall, & Walter Watts, eds., The Psychological Aspects of Abortion (Washington, DC: University Publications of America, 1979), p. 132.

35. Ann Saltenberger, Every Woman Has a Right to Know the Dangers of Legal Abortion (Glassboro, NJ: Air-Plus Enterprises, 1982), reports two studies that found sexual coldness expressed by 33 percent of women within nine months after their abortions, and an additional 14 percent developed sexual coldness four to five years later (p. 131).

36. Cf. the stories of various "aborted women" in David C. Reardon, Aborted Women (Westchester, IL: Crossway, 1987), pp. 305-310, 151-157.

37. Ann Saltenberger, Every Woman Has a Right to Know the Dangers of Legal Abortion (Glassboro, NJ: Air-Plus Enterprises, 1982), p. 132; Greenglass, "Therapeutic Abortion and Psychiatric Disturbance in Canadian Women," Canadian Psychiatric A.J., Vol. 21, 1976, p. 45, found a 3 percent suicide rate.

38. R.M. Pickering, "Relative Risks of Low Birthweight in Scotland, 1980-2," Journal of Epidemiology and Community Health, Vol. 41, June 1987, pp. 133-137.

39. The Knickerbocker Times, Albany, New York, December 6, 1963, as cited in Judie Brown, et al. Stop School-Based Sex Clinics (Stafford, VA: American Life League, 1987), pp. 7-8.

40. Family Practice News, December 15, 1977, as cited by Brown, ibid.

41. New York Times, June 12, 1981, as cited in Brown, ibid.

42. A. Pietronpinto, "A Survey on Contraceptive Analysis," Medical Aspects of Human Sexuality, May 1987, p. 147.

43. William Marsiglio, & Frank L. Mott, "The Impact of Sex Education on Sexual Activity, Contraceptive Use and Premarital Pregnancy Among American Teenagers," Family Planning Perspectives, Vol. 4 (4), July/August 1986, pp. 151-160.

44. National Research Council, "Risking the Future -- Adolescent Sexuality, Pregnancy, and Childbearing" (Washington, DC: National Academy Press, 1987), p. 165.

47-042 - 92 - 5

45. Deborah Ann Dawson, "The Effects of Sex Education on Adolescent Behavior," Family Planning Perspectives, Vol. 18 (4), July/August 1986, pp. 166, 168-169.

46. cf. Jacqueline R. Kasun, "Sex Education: The Hidden Agenda," The World & I, Vol. 4 (9), September 1989, p. 494f.

47. Donald P. Orr, Mary Beiter, & Gary Ingersoll, "Premature Sexual Activity as an Indicator of Psychosocial Risk," Pediatrics, Vol. 87 (2), February 1991, pp. 141-147; R. Jessor, & S.L. Jessor, Problem Behavior and Psychosocial Development: A Longitudinal Study of Youth (New York: Academic Press, 1977); J.E. Donovan, & R. Jessor, "Problem Drinking and the Dimensions of Involvement with Drugs: A Gutman Scalogram Analysis of Adolescent Drug Use," American Journal of Public Health, Vol. 73, 1983, pp. 543-552; F.L. Mott, & R.J. Haurin, "Linkages between Sexual Activity and Alcohol and Drug Use Among American Adolescents," Family Planning Perspectives, Vol. 20, 1988, pp. 128-136.

48. L.S. Zabin, "The Association between Smoking and Sexual Behavior among Teens in the United States Contraception Clinics," American Journal of Public Health, Vol. 74, 1984, pp. 261-262.

49. J.E. Donovan, & R. Jessor, "Structure of Problem Behavior in Adolescence and Young Adulthood," Journal of Consulting Clinical Psychology, Vol. 53, 1985, pp. 890-904; G.M. Ingersoll, & D.P. Orr, "Behavioral and Emotional Risk in Early Adolescents," Journal of Early Adolescence, Vol. 9, 1989, pp. 396-408; D.P. Orr, M. Beiter, & G. Ingersoll, "Premature Sexual Activity as an Indicator of Psychosocial Risk," Pediatrics, Vol. 87 (2), February 1991, pp. 141-147; A.R. Stiffman, F. Earls, L.N. Robins, K.G. Jung, & P. Kulbok, "Adolescent Sexual Activity and Pregnancy: Socio-Environmental Problems, Physical Health and Mental Health," Journal of Youth and Adolescence, Vol. 16, 1987, pp. 497-509; S.L. Jessor, & R. Jessor, "Transition from Virginity to Nonvirginity among Youth: A Socio-Psychological Study Over Time," Developmental Psychology, vol. 11, 1975, pp. 473-484.

50. Donald P. Orr, Mary Beiter, & Gary Ingersoll, "Premature Sexual Activity..."

51. D. Orr, M. Wilbrandt, C. Brach, S. Rauch, & G. Ingersoll, "Reported Sexual Behaviors and Self-Esteem among Young Adolescents," AJDC, Vol. 143, 1989, pp. 86-90.

52. Carol Tavris, & Susan Sadd, The Redbook Report on Female Sexuality (New York: Dell, 1977), pp. 74-76.

53. Travis & Sadd, p. 76.

54. Louis Harris and Associates, American Teens Speak: Sex, Myths, TV, and Birth Control (New York: Planned Parenthood Federation of America, 1986), p. 19.

55. Mark D. Hayward, & Junichi Yagi, "Contraceptive Failure in the United States: Estimates from the 1982 National Survey of Family Growth," Family Planning Perspectives, Vol. 18 (5), September/October 1986, table 5; Melvin Zelnik, Michael A. Koenig, & Kim J. Young, "Sources of Prescription Contraceptives and Subsequent Pregnancy Among Young Women," Family Planning Perspectives, Vol. 16 (1), January/February 1984, pp. 6-13.

56. Leslie V.H. Hill, et al., "Prevalence of Lower Genital Tract Infections in Pregnancy," Sexually Transmitted Diseases, Vol. 15, January-March 1988, pp. 5-10.

57. Leslie V.H. Hill, et al., ibid.

58. Asta Kenney, "School-Based Clinics: A National Conference," Family Planning Perspectives, Vol. 18 (1), January/February 1986, pp. 6, 28.

59. Nicholas J. Fiumara, "Effectiveness of Condoms in Preventing V.D.," New England Journal of Medicine, October 21, 1971, p. 972.

60. Peter Gotzsche, & Merete Hording, Scandanavian Journal of Infectious Disease. From the Department of Infectious Diseases., Rigshospitalet, Copenhagemn, Denmark, 20:233-234, 52, 1988. As cited in McDowell, The Myths of Sex Education.

61. D.R. Mishell, "Contraception," The New England Journal of Medicine, Vol. 320, 1989, pp. 777-787.

62. J. Mann, et al., "Condom Use and HIV Infection among Prostitutes in Zaire (letter)," The New England Journal of Medicine, Vol. 316, 1987, p. 345; M.A. Fischl, et al., "Evaluation of Heterosexual Partners, Children, and Household Contacts of Adults with AIDS," The Journal of the American Medical Association, Vol. 257, 1987, pp. 640-644; M.A. Fischl, & G.M. Dickinson, "Heterosexual Transmission of Acquired Immunodeficiency Syndrome (letter)," The Journal of the American Medical Association, Vol. 257, 1987, pp. 2288-2289.

63. Shepherd Smith, & Anita Moreland Smith, Christians in the Age of AIDS (Wheaton, IL: Victor, 1990), pp. 123-124.

64. Bruce Voeller, president of the Mariposa Foundation, noted that if the failure rate is 10 percent when condoms are used to prevent pregnancy, their failure rate for preventing AIDS would be considerably higher. In Bruce Voeller, & Malcolm Potts, British Medical Journal, October 26, 1986, p. 1196; and UPI story, "Condoms May Not Prevent AIDS Transfer, Expert Says," San Francisco

Examiner, November 7, 1985.

65. "Condoms: Experts Fear False Sense of Security," The New York Times, August 18, 1987.

66. Theresa Crenshaw, "Condom Advertising," testimony before the House Subcommittee on Health and the Environment, February 10, 1987, p. 2.

67. "Condoms: Experts Fear False Sense of Security," The New York Times, August 18, 1987.

68. "Condoms: Experts Fear False Sense of Security," The New York Times, August 18, 1987.

69. Telephone interview, September 1, 1987, as cited in Jo Ann Gasper, ed., What you Need to Know About AIDS (Ann Arbor, MI: Servant, 1990), p. 64.

70. "Koch Orders New AIDS Ads Stressing Sexual Abstinence," The New York Times, June 8, 1987.

71. The Department of Health and Human Services (HHS) writes,

> You should store condoms in a cool, dry place out of direct sunlight, perhaps in a drawer or closet. If you want to keep one with you, put it in a loose pocket, wallet or purse for no more than a few hours at a time. Extreme termperature - espectially heat - can make latex brittle or gummy (like an old balloon). So, don't keep these latex products in a hot place like a glove compartment (Condoms and Sexually Transmitted Diseases...Especially AIDS, HHS Publication FDA90-4239).

Yet Richard Smith points out that the average time for distribution is 25 days. During this time condoms are subjected to the most extreme temperatures and conditions, all of which decrease the condoms' chance of effectiveness (Richard Smith, "The Condom: Is It Really Safe" (Public Eduction Committee, P.O. Box 33082, Seattle, WA, 1990).

The Washington Post pointed out the dangers to such practices for product liability:

> Under new concepts of product liability, they have been awarding huge judgments to compensate victims of "wrongful birth", even when there was no negligence in the conventional sense.... Manufacturers ... have withdrawn all but one minor brand of IUD from the market, and almost entirely suspended US research on new contraceptive products... Condoms are not foolproof either, and even if one in 10 million sold leads to a

> wrongful death AIDS verdict, their price will rise out of reach of many users, with incalculable consequences for public health (September 29, 1987).

Likewise, it appears that public service announcements that advertize "safe sex" or "protected sex" could be subject to action, since they are false and misleading due to the "clear and present danger" that exists for STDs and death.

Disclaimers are no longer safe havens of immunity. According to a recent New Jersey Supreme Court ruling, tobacco companies still face liability suits from smokers despite health warnings on cigarette packs (Dewey v R.J. Reynolds Tobacco Co, July 26, 1990). Some who became infected with AIDS after a blood tranfusion are also winning claims against blood banks which gave them the infected blood (cf. Blood Bank Week, Vol. 7 (12), March 23, 1990).

When the public health establishment endorses defective products, Smith cites a host of cases that suggest they too are liable (pp. 58-101). After reading his study, health officials and county lawyers in Burlington County, New Jersey decided it would be unwise to distribute condoms as part of their AIDS education program.

72. John O.G. Billy, "Effects of Sexual Activity on Adolescent Social and Psychological Development," Social Psychology Quarterly, Vol. 51, 1988, pp. 190-212.

73. Richard R. Troiden, & Margaret P. Jendrek, "Does Sexual Ideology Correlate with Level of Sexual Experience? Assessing the Construct Validity of the SAS," The Journal of Sex Research, Vol. 23 (2), May 1987, pp. 256-261; Emogene Fox, & Michael Young, "Religiosity, Sex Guilt, and Sexual Behavior Among College Students," Health Values, Vol. 13, March/April 1989, pp. 32-37.

74. Edward M. Levine, & Eugene J. Kanin, "Sexual Violence Among Dates and Acquaintances: Trends and Their Implications for Marriage and Family," Journal of Family Violence, Vol. 2 (1), 1987, pp. 55-65.

75. William Marsiglio, "Adolescent Fathers in the United States: Their Initial Living Arrangements, Marital Experience and Educational Outcomes," Family Planning Perspectives, Vol. 19 (6), November/December 1987, pp. 240-251.

76. Kristin A. Moore, Christine W. Nord, & James L. Peterson, "Nonvoluntary Sexual Activity Among Adolescents," Family Planning Perspectives, Vol. 21 (3), May/June 1989, pp. 110-114.

77. Raymond A. Knight, & Robert A. Prentky, "The Developmental Antecedents and Adult Adaptations of Rapist Subtypes," Criminal Justice and Behavior, Vol. 14, December 1987, pp. 403-426.

78. Brent C. Miller, & C. Raymond Bingham, "Family Configuration in Relation to the Sexual Behavior of Female Adolescents," Journal of Marriage and the Family, Vol. 51, 1989, pp. 499-506; Susan Newcomer, & J. Richard Udry, "parental Marital Status Effects on Adolescent Sexual Behavior," Journal of Marriage and the Family, Vol. 49 (2), May 1987, pp. 235-240; Robert L. Flewelling, & Karl E. Bauman, "Family Structure as a Predictor of Initial Substance Abuse and Sexual Intercourse in Early Adolescence," Journal of Marriage and the Family, Vol. 52, 1990, pp. 171-181; Suzanne Riggs, Anthony J. Alario, & Colleen McHorney, "Health Risk Behaviors and Attempted Suicide in Adolescents Who Report Prior Maltreatment," The Journal of Pediatrics, Vol. 116, 1990, pp. 815-821; Denise Kandel, & Emily Rosenbaum, "Early Onset of Adolescent Sexual Behavior and Drug Involvement," Journal of Marriage and the Family, Vol. 52, 1990, pp. 783-898.

Joyce White also found that young women who live in intact families and who are engaging in premarital sex, postpone their use of contraceptives longer than those who do not live in intact family. She ignores, however, the increased sexual activity among these teens. Joyce E. White, "Influence of Parents, Peers, and Problem-Solving on Contraceptive Use," Pediatric Nursing, Vol. 13, September/October 1987, pp. 317-321.

79. Joseph W. Scott, & Robert Perry, "Black Family Headship Structure, Parent-Child Affect, Communication, and Delaying Teenage Pregnancy," National Journal of Sociology, Vol. 4, 1990, pp. 63-80.

80. Karen Lee Fingerman, "Sex and the Working Mother: Adolescent Sexuality, Sex Role Typing and Family Background," Adolescence, Vol. 93, 1989, pp. 1-15.

81. Brent C. Miller, et al., "Family Configuration and Adolescent Sexual Attitudes and Behavior," Population and Environment: Behavioral and Social Issues, Vol. 9, Summer 1987, pp. 111-123.

82. Suzanne Southworth, & J. Conrad Schwarz, "Post-Divorce Contact, Relationship with Father, and Heterosexual Trust in Female College Students," American Journal of Orthopsychiatry, Vol. 57 (3), July 1987, pp. 379-381.

83. Katherine F. Darabi, & Vilma Ortiz, "Childbearing Among Young Latino Women in the United States," American Journal of Public Health, Vol. 77 (1), January 1987, pp. 25-28.

84. Jacqueline Kasun, "Sex Education: A New Philosophy for America?," The Family in America, July 1989, p. 4; Robert H. DuRant, Robert Pendergast, & Carolyn Seymore, "Sexual Behavior Among Hispanic Female Adolescents in the United States," Pediatrics, Vol. 85, 1990, pp. 1051-1058.

85. Carol S. Aneshensel, "Onset of Fertility-Related Events During Adolescence: A Prospective Comparison of Mexican American and Non-Hispanic White Females," American Journal of Public Health, Vol. 80, 1990, pp. 959-963.

86. Craig St. John, & David Rowe, "Adolescent Background and Fertility Norms: Implications for Racial Differences in Early Childbearing," Social Science Quarterly, Vol. 71, 1990, pp. 152-162.

87. Office of Population Affairs, The Adolescent Family Life Demonstration Projects, pp. 242-246; Terrance Olson, & Christopher Wallace, "A Sampler of AANCHOR" (Provo, Utah: Brigham Young University), p. 35.

88. The Teen-Aid Family Life Education Project, an Evaluation Report prepared for the Office of Adolescent Pregnancy Program (OAPP) by the Institute for Research and Evaluation, December 28, 1988. Stan E. Weed, Joseph A. Olsen, and Raja Tanas, Project Evaluators.

89. UPI release, January 12, 1988, and studies complied by Project Respect for the second-year pilot program. Similar results are available for the third year.

90. Letter from Joe DeDiminicantanio to LeAnna Benn, October 2, 1987, cited in Dinah Richard, Has Sex Education Failed Our Teenagers? (Pomona, CA: Focus on the Family, 1990), p. 60.

91. "Teen Choice Project Evaluation: Interim Evaluation Report," draft, July 18, 1988, as cited in Dinah Richard, Has Sex Education Failed Our Teenagers?, p. 60.

Chairwoman SCHROEDER. Thank you very much.

I think we will start with the questioning, and because of the time constraints, if we can hold our questions to five minutes, it could be helpful.

Congressman Wolf.

Mr. WOLF. Thank you very much, Madam Chair.

There are so many questions you could ask that five minutes will not do it. So maybe we will come back around or maybe we will not have the time.

I have a whole series of questions I am just going to submit for the record. If you all can comment; it does seem to me that there are diametrically different opinions among Dr. Hayton, Dr. Lyons, Ms. Mayden, and Dr. Selverstone.

Doctor Hayton, you make, I think, a very telling point, which came up again yesterday which I was not, quite frankly, aware of, and that is the failure rate with regard to condoms. Of course, if they do fail, we may very well be destining an individual to death because there is no cure with regard to HIV.

Are there studies or should there be additional studies so we can reconcile the differences? And perhaps, Ms. Mayden, you can answer this, too. Do you both agree that we should be doing more studies in the area of condom failure to see if the figures are as accurate as you say not only with regard to pregnancy, but with regard to disease and, secondly, more studies with regard to the question of abstinence?

Maybe you could both answer that question.

Dr. HAYTON. Yes, you know, I totally agree. The best study and one of the few studies on HIV with the use of condoms showed an 18 percent failure rate, and that was with married partners who were adults, using condoms, not teenagers using condoms.

Mr. WOLF. Who did that study?

Dr. HAYTON. Which is drastically different, and 18 percent failure rate is drastic. So much more research needs to be done, especially with teenagers, but it is difficult.

Mr. WOLF. But who did the study? Can you tell us?

Dr. HAYTON. I know I have it cited.

Mr. WOLF. If you can submit it for the record.

Dr. HAYTON. Yes.

No. 62 in my footnotes M.A. Fischal, et al., "Evaluation of Heterosexual Partners, Children, and Household Contracts of Adults with AIDS, "The Journal of the American Medical Association, Vol. 257, 1987, pp. 640–644; M.A. Fischal, & G.M. Dickinson, Heterosexual Transmission of Acquired Immunodeficiency Syndrome (letter)," The Journal of the American Medical Association, Vol. 257, 1987, pp. 2288–2289.

Mr. WOLF. Ms. Mayden.

Ms. MAYDEN. Part of the failure rate, I think, with condoms is that they are used incorrectly, and one of the things that we do in the Three for Free Program——

[Applause.]

Ms. MAYDEN [continuing]. Is provide information in terms of the correct usage of condoms. I mean we all think that, you know, I guess, because you are male, you are born knowing how to put on a condom, but unfortunately what we are finding, particularly with teenagers, is that there is incorrect usage.

The other thing I would like to point out to you——

Mr. WOLF. But the question is do you believe there should be additional studies to reconcile the differences with regard to condom failure, with regard to pregnancies, and with regard to diseases?

And, secondly, do you think there should be additional studies, although there may be differences, with regard to the question of abstinence?

Ms. MAYDEN. I am not so sure we need additional studies. The reason I say that is the Surgeon General has come out in his goals for the nation for the year 2000. He has very clearly put out one of his goals—to increase condom usage by doubling it in the nation, and I think if our Surgeon General is giving us this information and saying that, this is one of the ways that he——

Mr. WOLF. No, I understand that. I agree, but the question is do you think there should be additional scientific research, not philosophical or political, discussions, but scientific research both on the failure rate with regard to pregnancies and the failure rate with regard to disease to see if Mr. Hayton is right, and also on the question of abstinence so that you can come at this from both ends? Do you agree or disagree that there should be more research?

Ms. MAYDEN. I think that is fine if people want to put money in research. I think money ought to go into services.

Mr. WOLF. Well, I know. I agree. The government has gotten involved in many things, and you do not want to just pour money down a rat hole if it is not working. If it is working, fine, but there may be a varied opinion.

Dr. Lyons, do you have any comment on that?

Dr. LYONS. Yes. My primary area of research is in serious mental illness, and routinely in that area, they take various proposed treatments and compare them to each other to see which works, and what I find kind of surprising about this particular literature is that has not been done, and I do not understand why.

I would suggest that if we really want to understand what works and what does not, take the various proposed interventions and compare them to each other in a nice, random assignment, experimental way that could really give us an answer so that we could put the money where it belongs in services.

But from my perspective in reading the literature and understanding it, I think teenage pregnancy is a multi-caused social problem. There are all sorts of social and economic factors that lead our teenagers to more and more become pregnant. I do not think failure of contraception is one of those problems.

And to address the problem as a treatment by providing contraception does not get at the root cause. It is like putting a Bandaid on a bullet wound, and it is not that it is right or wrong. It just does not work, and that is what I think.

Mr. WOLF. Well, I want to thank you all, and I am not taking issue. I think, if anything, the differences between Dr. Lyons and Ms. Mayden and Dr. Hayton is the lack of certainty. Although each side may be very certain, we really do need more data and more information.

I suggest research ought to be done by the Public Health Service and by the Food and Drug Administration and by agencies of the government with credible people who have no ax to grind on either side so that we truly can know because if you are giving out faulty condoms to an individual, you may be sentencing that individual to death.

The other question, and I know my time is running out, if you can submit for the record: have there been any lawsuits in this area? You just alluded to it.

I did want to make two last comments, if I can with the chair. Mr. Walker, I want to congratulate you and Burtrell Selph. There is a young man in my office who has been trying to urge us to do the same thing, in Northern Virginia and I am meeting with Mayor Dixon on Thursday, and I am going to tell her about your program.

Andy Hart, who works in my office, has mentioned your program to me. He said it is one of the most successful going and has encouraged us to adopt it in the Washington, D.C. area. I am going to ask Mayor Dixon, if you can give us your telephone number, to have someone follow up with you because I think that your program is very successful.

In the District of Columbia, there is a lack of police athletic leagues. There are very, very few ball fields, and I think what you say is so true and good, and we would like to follow up with that.

My comment for the record, and I will elaborate a little bit, is I guess the one important issue coming from the testimony, and I am glad that Dr. Hayton mentioned it, is about values. Values, values. I am a little bit concerned, Ms. Mayden, that there may be an opportunity for a young child in a school-based health clinic who cannot get two aspirins from the nurse, but is able to get birth control pills or condoms.

And the role of parental involvement. I mean you want to know who your children are with, who they are talking to and who they are getting things from. I just think to have a value-free philosophy is wrong. I am not suggesting what you are doing is value-free. I realize we really have not had an opportunity to get into this.

I mean I do not want to be a wet blanket at the party, but there are some things that are right, and there are some things that are wrong. I think what you are doing, and I might say your figures for Baltimore on the gonorrhea study are quite impressive, and I commend you for them. I am not taking issue, but there are some things that are right and wrong.

Just to dispense, I would ask the chair if we could have a hearing on the value question and values.

Chairwoman SCHROEDER. Does the gentleman think the chair does not have values?

Mr. WOLF. No.

Chairwoman SCHROEDER. Oh, okay.

Mr. WOLF. No, let the record show that I do not feel that way, and if I said anything that would infer that.

What I wanted to do was ask the chair to have a hearing on values. Congressman Hastert had raised the question of having a hearing on values and instilling values. If I inferred that the chair did not have values, I do apologize.

Chairwoman SCHROEDER. Okay, and could I call time to let Congresswoman Collins ask a few questions? The bells have gone off.

Mr. WOLF. I thank you very much, and I will submit some questions for them.

Chairwoman SCHROEDER. Congresswoman Collins.

Ms. COLLINS. Thank you, Madam Chair.

I am going to run through my list real quickly and maybe any responses can be given to the record.

For Dr. Selverstone, his statistics that 80 percent of young people waited in our day and age for marriage, I just wonder if they waited or if they did not tell. [Laughter.]

I am very serious about this, now, very serious because we are about the same age, and I wonder also if 80 percent of women waited and 80 percent of men, or did 80 percent of women wait and 20 percent of men.

So I think those are very interesting questions that if you can respond to the record, I would appreciate that.

To Dr. Hayton and Dr. Lyons, I wonder if you put too much responsibility on the school-based clinic to solve a lot of ills of society. It is very difficult for school-based clinics, health clinics to stop or diminish teenage sexual activity and to increase the sanctity of marriage when you have open sex on TV and in the movies all day long.

When I look at a movie, I see naked bodies. On TV, prime time, eight o'clock, naked bodies having sexual activity. I know people do not like censorship, but how in the world can a condom, a little latex condom, fight against these beautiful people, beautiful people on TV showing you that sex, a horrible kind of sex to me, is a good thing to do if you want to be a beautiful person.

It seems to me that you are putting too much responsibility—your statistics are probably true that sexual activity increases, but I would not put the increase to the health clinic. I would put it to society that sells toilet tissue with a woman's body on TV. You know, they have a woman in a robe coming out of the shower, and it is some kind of a soft touch toilet tissue.

So teenagers are very susceptible. People tell me that sex and violence in the movies and on TV has nothing to do with the murder rate or the sexual activity, but if it is good enough to sell cars and gym shoes and cereal, you cannot tell me that it is not also selling sexual promiscuity.

Dr. HAYTON. Good Congresswoman, the way they do research is to use pretests and postests, and they try to control for other factors in the environment. They put certain people in control groups that are not in—I did not study school-based health clinics. It was condom-based sex education programs—they would put some people in a sex ed. program and some people not in a sex ed. program, and then they would control for other factors: socio-economic factors, for example just to try to just get, and granted sometimes they are off, but probably all kids in both groups would be watching the TV and, you know, doing normal kinds of things, going to school, etc. The goal of these studies is to try to just find the specific effectiveness of the school based program or the sex ed. condom-based program or any other kind of treatment program.

That way they would see what that program does to that adolescent, and the research consistently shows it does have certain effects, but the effects are not the ones that were desired.

Ms. COLLINS. Also——

Dr. LYONS. Could I have the floor for a second? Could I respond to that also?

Ms. COLLINS. Okay.

Dr. LYONS. Yes, I would agree with you completely that there is a large number of causes, or at least up to a point, I think. There is a large number of causes that are influencing the problem, and that the solution to the problem is focusing on the causes, and that is where I think our limited resources should go.

Ms. COLLINS. Okay. I also wonder if sex education classes make the teenage girl more apt to talk about what she is doing, more able to communicate the activity that is going on. Dr. Selverstone?

Dr. SELVERSTONE. We consistently see that. Invariably the young people in the courses, whether it is a group for high school or whether it is middle school children talking with their parents. Invariably they say that the mere presence of a sexuality education program legitimizes conversation about sexuality, and I think that the feedback that I get is that it legitimizes it so that young people can talk about it.

There are young people, young women, in our course who have said, "I am so glad I had this course. It let me know that I can be 18 years old and still a virgin and that is okay." And what it does is it empowers—I will use the same word that was used before—it says: you have a legitimate right to talk about what your needs are and what your wants are, and you do not have to do something just because somebody asks you to, but you need to learn how to negotiate whatever behavior in which you are going to engage.

Ms. COLLINS [presiding]. Well, do we have to vote now? All right. Then as a temporary chair then, I would like to recess this hearing for a few minutes until Mrs. Schroeder comes back, and we will run across the street and vote.

Thank you all very much. And I want to tell you Ms. Toure is gone, but Ms. Toure and Mr. Walker have been very inspirational, hearing your comments. I think when all is said and done, the message is going to have to be given at the grassroots level and any changes will be done in the community by community folk, and it will be up to the experts to research and study those and publish what is being done so that others perhaps can emulate them.

I want to thank you all very much and ask if you will have the patience to wait for the chair to come back. Thank you.

[Recess.]

Chairwoman SCHROEDER. The chair tried not to ask questions so other Members could ask their questions and move on, but I thought there were a few things that we needed to fill in on.

Obviously, as I said, Mr. Walker, we think you are fantastic, and we want to see you in Denver, too. So let us get the information, and we really salute what you are doing.

Dr. Selverstone, I wanted to ask if you wanted to comment on anything you heard from the rest of the panel. I think for two days we have heard two conflicting views. One is we should deal directly with teens, and the other is we are inciting teens to action if we deal directly, and that part of the high incidence or the high increase of sexual activity has been because of dealing more directly with teens.

You started out by saying the problem with my generation versus the new generation is that the numbers have so shifted, from 20–80 to 80–20. Has anyone figured out what is causing this? I mean, can you be of any help in documenting that?

Dr. SELVERSTONE. Indeed, I think there are probably a variety. The hormones are the same. We know that the physiology has not changed, and probably in most ways the psychology has not changed, and what has changed is the sociology, and I think what we need to do, therefore, is to have an impact on part of that sociology.

I am intrigued that we teach civics every year from kindergarten through the 12th grade, American history and government, and so forth, and we have abysmal failures. Only 50 percent of our adults go to the polls, and the truth is I think that 50 percent of those who vote vote wrong, and that means we have a 75 percent failure rate, and nobody seriously suggests that we stop civics education.

What we say is we need to do a better job of this, and I think we need to really be aware that there are very powerful forces going on in our society that are impelling our young people to dangerous activities, and it is not just sexuality. It is alcohol and drugs and suicide and underachievement in school and eating disorders and exploitation in sexism and racism, and the whole variety.

I think research tends to suggest that the key issue has to do with developmental tasks and helping young people develop a sense of their own identity and their sense of connectedness with other people and of their own power, that they are in charge of their own lives.

I think what we discover when young people get pregnant prematurely is they have given up on that. Those are youngsters who say, "I have no control over my life. Nothing good will happen to me anyway," and I guess it is Leon Dash, the newspaper writer in Washington who wrote a book on children who want to have children, and a recent AP, I think, article yesterday starts to talk about that, that there is some significant number of young people who, indeed, get pregnant because they wish to.

So I think what we need to do is recognize that this is an enormously diverse society in which we are living, and that any one program or any uni-dimensional program is not going to be successful.

I think the advantage of working with parents is each parent can help share their values with their own child and not just "this is what I believe," but "this is why I believe it, how I got to that point of view."

The schools are one place and the youth-serving agencies perhaps are the second place where youngsters can try to make sense out of it; that a kid can say, in contradistinction to Representative Wolf—I disagree that we have a clear sense of right and wrong—that with Judaism the Orthodox say homosexuality is a sin, and the Reformed Jews now ordain gay and lesbian rabbis.

Certainly what we have seen in the Episcopal and Presbyterian Church documents recently about sexuality suggests that there is, indeed, no clear sense of right and wrong on such very basic issues.

The responsibility of schools and really appropriate parents, I think, is to help young people make sense out of this. If the media says this and the President says this and my clergy says this and my mother says this, but my divorced father says that and my peers say this—each of which is different—then how do I make sense out of that?

What we really need to do is not only develop good curriculum and do it comprehensively K–12, but we need to invest lots of money in teacher training. The Guttmacher Institute says there are 50,000 people out there teaching about sexuality, and for about 45,000 of them, this is simply a part-time thing that they do. They are physical educators who are teaching one class. They are school nurses who are teaching one class. They are science teachers who teach a little biology.

And what we really need to do is to get teachers who can really talk with young people, who feel comfortable about sexuality, who have a mental health perspective, and say, to students "This is a very key part of you. We all have different values, and I will help you learn how to weigh that and to consider that and make decisions in your best interest."

A little piece that I wanted to say about the controversy and effectiveness of condoms. Interesting research by Robert Hatcher, who is by all reputes perhaps the expert on reproductive technology, and one of the research studies that he cites is that among reproductive health people, the failure rate of condoms was one in 161. Among teenagers and people in clinics, it was one in 16, and among college educated adults, it was one in 92.

What that suggests is that the condom does not change. The way people use it changes, and we need to educate people about how to use it properly so that they know, for example, that petroleum-based lubricants will eat away at a condom. That is education, and that is the whole difference between ineffective use of whatever the reproductive technology is and effective use of that.

Chairwoman SCHROEDER. All very interesting points.

The Congressional Caucus on Women's Issues has been studying our total lack of looking at research on contraceptive devices. I mean the administration has just totally deferred, and this country really has done none in the last I do not know how many years.

There is a gentleman at Johns Hopkins who has a very interesting contraceptive device that it appears women can use that is very good at preventing disease, but is unable to get administration funding for it, and of course, they have been trying to get funding for better forms of condoms, safer forms and so forth.

Is there anyone at the table that would object to that? That certainly makes some sense, that you give people more user-friendly or more options. Does anybody object to that type?

Dr. LYONS. Yes, if I could take the opportunity to respond, first of all, I would like to take a little umbrage to your initial reinterpretation of my testimony that I was saying that being direct incites teenagers. That is not at all what the data that I have presented to this committee shows.

It shows that the provision of contraceptives does not prevent births.

In terms of contraception technology, I think that is great. I think that the work at Johns Hopkins is important. I think that the better the contraceptives work, the happier people will be in terms of their family planning.

But I also would go back to what Dr. Selverstone said, that education is also very important, but education is a stage phenomenon. You do not teach people how to divide until they know how to multiply. You do not teach people how to multiply until they know how to subtract. You do not teach people how to subtract until you teach them how to add.

And I think the big controversy is where in the educational system different levels of education about sexuality is important. As a clinical psychologist, I have worked in sex therapy teaching couples how to have intimate, satisfying sexual relations and orgasm, and so forth. I think that is important, but I think that is important at a different life stage than I think other members of this committee think.

Chairwoman SCHROEDER. I guess I am troubled because I think we have mixed the terms so much, that anyone reading this hearing will get very confused.

There are the sexuality courses, and there are many of them still in this country that were exactly like the ones I had when I was in school where they pulled the chart down over the black board, and it was like a plumbing course. You know, this is how this works, and that is how that works, and that was the end of it.

It gave you no information on how to deal with your own emotions. So if that is what we mean by sexuality courses, I can understand that if you are giving out contraceptives, if you are doing anything, you still kind of walk away not having a feeling of empowerment as to what you do.

And then there are the more holistic approaches, which I think Ms. Mayden is talking about, where you try to really put in the whole scope and include the parents and then contraceptives fall into their own place in that whole range.

I mean that certainly would be much more what I would endorse, and my guess then is that if you had all of the programs like that, you would have different kinds of statistics to talk about.

Dr. LYONS. That is certainly possible. Those programs have not existed or have not been studied. As I was telling Mr. Walker at the break, I think his program has a better chance of preventing teenage pregnancies than all of the condoms in Chicago. I think that is exactly the kind of thing. It is getting at the root cause of the problem.

It is value based. It is teaching important things.

Chairwoman SCHROEDER. I would like to have both Mr. Walker or Mr. Selph talk a bit about young males in the program. I thought that their posters that they had from Baltimore were very interesting about how you get more male responsibility into this.

Mr. WALKER. I think, Congresswoman Schroeder, that, again, basketball is just a hook. Okay. Value systems are so important. What we try and do is we are trying to undergird what manhood really means, and I think that that is where the emphasis should be put.

It just seems to me that I learned at an early age back in the second grade. I can remember how the physical education teacher—we had a dance unit, if you will—and at that time, all the physical education classes were second graders. The girls were on one side. The boys were on the other side, and it was a dance unit, and I can remember Coach Red Tandy telling us, "I am going to show you how to ask the ladies to dance," and the curtain raised up, and 50 little girls on one side and 50 little guys on the other side, and he told us in the locker room prior to coming out there that you walk up to a young lady. You ask her, "May I have this dance?"

If she says no, that is okay. Still feel good about yourself because she may not want to dance with you. Ask someone else, but meander around. That is how I knew in the second grade what the word "meander" meant, and ask someone else because no woman wants to be second.

So of course, the curtain goes up. No one wants to make the first move, and I made the mistake of making eye contact with Coach Tandy. He told me to go over there and make my move, and I did, and of course, the young lady I asked said no.

So I had to walk all the way back to the other side of the room. Everyone just burst out with laughter, but in any case, that broke the ice, and everyone had a good time.

When we got back in the locker room, at that particular time Coach Tandy says, "Gil Walker, stand up. You did an excellent job, and you always will be okay about yourself, and you never will have any problems with women," and to this day I do not. [Laughter.]

But the point that I am trying to make is I learned that in the second grade. These young men that we are dealing with, no one ever took the opportunity to tell them about personal hygiene, about how to treat and respect a woman, about how to feel good about yourself.

So what I submit to you and to everyone else on this panel, that contraceptives, I think they will work, but the first thing is you have got to have some type of respect and dignity for the person that you are dealing with. Then you all can talk together about how to put a contraceptive on and how to use it and that type of thing.

In our particular community, that is a problem. Men do not know how to be men. Making babies is not being a man. Taking care of babies is.

So because we have their attention with this basketball program, not only I, but other guys who come in and do mandatory workshops at the end of each basketball game that talk about life; we talk about AIDS; we talk about sex education; we talk about employment; we talk about all these things that go into making responsible individuals, and I think that is the key, the value system.

You know, I like wearing gold, but your gold is no good to me if I have got to take it from around your neck. That is the thing that we are putting back to these young men in public housing, and it is working.

Chairwoman SCHROEDER. Very good.

Mr. Selph, what do you find among your peers?

Mr. SELPH. Well, what I find among my peers is different gang members being able to relate to each other. It had not been that way until Midnight Basketball has come along. Different gang members would be sitting here at this table, and there would be, you know, words flying back at each other, and maybe the police would have to come in.

As far as myself, I have had a strong based family, you know, that supported me, and you know, I am grateful for that. And when I got involved with Midnight Basketball, it seems like Gil Walker took me up under his wing, and I have learned a lot of things, and I have done a lot of things that I probably would not have done without Midnight Basketball.

The men in Midnight Basketball also look up to Gil Walker as a father figure, and they do what he says because they know if they do not do what he says, they are out of the program, and you really do not want to go up against Mr. Walker, or Commissioner Walker as you please, because he will chew you out real quick, and that gives everyone in the league of, you know, self-improvement. You want to do for yourself as well as to please Commissioner Walker.

So that is the big thing in the Midnight Basketball League.

Chairwoman SCHROEDER. Well, that is very, very impressive.

Well, I thank you all for staying. I am sorry we kept you all so long. I am sure that there will be more things. If more things occur to you, again, the record will be open for two weeks before we close it out and print it, and I thank you.

Oh, I am sorry. Yes, Barbara is back.

Ms. COLLINS. Thank you.

Chairwoman SCHROEDER. Thank you for taking over as I ran over. Excuse me. We will not close now. I am really pleased to have Ms. Collins back, and if you have some questions.

Ms. COLLINS. I asked all of my questions while you were gone. So I thank you.

I thank the panel very much. I think this is such an important topic that needs to be discussed on the congressional level, and hopefully we can get some messages back home to the people.

Madam Chair, I pointed out that we cannot really expect school-based health clinics and condoms to make up for all of the media, TV and movies, encouragement of sex or premarital sex, and we just have a big job ahead of us.

Thank you all very much.

Chairwoman SCHROEDER. I think you make a very good point. We were pointing out yesterday, too, that the alcohol industry has almost taken over sports. If you watch anything on TV, you are just inundated with that, and you are inundated with sex. And that is such a pervasive influence in our culture that even if parents are having good dialogue with kids, the idea that it would be wonderful if we could return to the world as it was when we were growing up and did not have it, is not going to happen because TV is there every day. And we just have to deal with the kind of realistic pressure that are being put on them.

So I think that is a very good point.

Well, thank you all again very much for being here, and with that we adjourn the hearing.

[Whereupon, at 12:46 p.m., the select committee was adjourned.]

[Material submitted for inclusion in the record follows:]

Prepared Statement of Congresswoman Joan Kelly Horn, a Representative In Congress From the State of Missouri

I want to welcome all of you here today. I am very impressed by the line-up.

It is very important that we involve the adolescents themselves in the strategy and program design of our youth programs. We are learning that now through experience. The programs that seem to work the best are the ones that give "ownership" of the adolescents feelings, needs and desires back to the adolescent. Young people must know they can control their own lives. It is often this lack of control that they are running from when they put themselves in risky situations.

I am not an expert on this subject, but I do have some experience working through the problems of youth. I am the mother of six children, and I struggled through many stressful times as a single mother. I was also a teacher and a public administrator before I came to Congress last year. All of these roles play a part in the everyday lives of our adolescents. I appreciate this opportunity to participate in finding solutions to these important problems.

Yesterday the Committee heard from academics and administrators about how we should approach the many problems facing our young people. Their excellent testimony presents a diversity of sound programs to reach out to our troubled adolescents and, actually, all our young people—because the risks of HIV infection, teen pregnancy, and drug and alcohol abuse cut across all boundaries.

In preparing for this hearing, I looked at the programs in my District that have evolved over the years to help address the problems of our youth. I say to them, as I can say to all of you here today, I am very impressed and you are doing a commendable job.

One point came through so clearly to me in this review and that was the gap—the lack of attention—between the ages of around 14–17 in youth programs. Not so surprisingly, this is time when our children are increasingly confronted with high risk situations. We need to find some alternative activities for that age group—like the midnight basketball program in Chicago, the theater program we saw here today, and drug- and alcohol-free dances. Maybe then we won't be forced to seek transitional housing for youths who have run away or been brought into the legal system because of criminal behavior.

Finally, we need a systematic approach to prevent crisis situations. We need a network in our communities that sits down and understands the pressures on our families that may lead to violence, addictions and other dysfunctional behaviors. The programs back in my District, in St. Louis and St. Charles County, have involved the adolescents in this process.

Kids will listen to other kids before they will listen to adults. The sooner we recognize that, the sooner we can move onto giving them the tools and the guidance for healthy behavior.

Again, I commend all of you here and applaud your efforts. I look forward to working together with you all.

PREPARED STATEMENT OF MERCEDES ARZU WILSON, PRESIDENT, FAMILY OF THE AMERICAS FOUNDATION, INC., MANDEVILLE, LA

Family of the Americas Foundation (FAF) is a non-profit organization incorporated in 1977, with its international headquarters in Maryland. FAF's purpose is to promote family unity by encouraging parents to meet their mutual responsibilities to each other and to their children. The programs of FAF instruct, educate, and counsel families in an effort to strengthen family traditions and promote responsible parenthood. We have conducted these programs in over 100 countries around the world, including the People's Republic of China.

Family of the Americas conducted a demonstration project from 1983 to 1987 called "Fertility Appreciation for Families". The project was funded by the U.S. Department of Health and Human Services under the Adolescent Family Life Act. We designed and thoroughly tested a unique family-centered sexuality program in New Orleans, LA, Charleston, SC, Wichita, KS and Corpus Christi, TX, which gave children the priceless gifts of understanding and appreciating sexuality as a normal, joyful and integral part of their human growth and development. It taught them that sexual intimacy is meant for the lifelong commitment of marriage between man and woman.

Reports from the four project sites indicated that, since its inception, the Fertility Appreciation for Families Project directly reached approximately 2,478 parent/adult participants and 3,678 adolescents. The program also had an indirect impact on the more than 5,000 children of the parent participants. Since the project ended four years ago, these children have been experiencing the benefits of the increased knowledge and communication skills of their parents.

These benefits were measured in the following way:

a. Demographic information forms were completed by approximately one-half of the program participants -- 1,412 parents/adults and 1750 adolescents (see Table I below).

TABLE I

Family of the Americas Foundation

Program for Families

Age Group	Number
Parent/AdultParticipants	2478
AdolescentParticipants	3678
Children of Parent Participants	5096

Participant by Race

White	50%
Black	7%
Hispanic	39%
NativeAmerican	2%
Asian	2%
Other	1%

b. Based on the data collected from these forms, an evaluation and summary of the project was drawn up by two professors at the University of New Orleans. At the end of the Study, the evaluators concluded that the majority of parents responding to the Communication Skills questionnaire agreed that they had become more confident in their ability to discuss sexual concerns with their children following the workshops, and that they would likely engage in such discussions more frequently than prior to the workshops. Adolescents tended to perceive their parents as better sources of information regarding sexual matters than they were prior to program participation. Furthermore, responses of both parents and adolescents to pre- and post-project discussion forms indicated that the frequency of parent/adolescent conversations concerning human sexuality had increased subsequent to training.

c. Ninety-three percent of all parents interviewed reported feeling comfortable discussing sexual concerns with their children, and 97.2% said they were confident in their knowledge of sexual information. Adolescents also reported continued confidence (81.3%). A comparison of teenage pregnancies among adolescents in the United States showed that Fertility Appreciation for Families program participants had a significantly lower pregnancy rate compared to other major studies (see Table II below):

TABLE II
COMPARISON OF STUDIES ON EFFECTIVENESS OF
FAMILY PLANNING PROGRAMS TO REDUCE TEENAGE PREGNANCY

STUDY	NUMBER OF TEENAGERS AGE 15-19 WITH PREGNANCIES
Alan Guttmacher Institute Study Statistics	96 per 1,000
Planned Parenthood Clinic Program (Weed and Olsen, 1986)	113 per 1,000
Family of the Americas Foundation (Evaluation Report, 1986)	5 per 1,000

Note: Data are from the Alan Guttmacher Institute Statistics & the National Center for Health Statistics, 1980 for national rate.

Our program shows immense potential in helping adolescents avoid sexual relations until marriage. If applied on a large scale basis, this project will have a major impact on the problem of sexual education for adolescents.

RECOMMENDATIONS

With all this evidence before the American people and before this committee, I strongly recommend that the government stop isolating the parents in this critical challenge of raising their children as responsible adults. It is a strange society indeed, where we teach that killing and stealing and drug abuse are wrong for teenagers, but that sexual promiscuity is permissible so long as they are protected. Protected from what, may I ask -- venereal disease? rape? violence? AIDS? abortion? The fact is -- none of the above!

The only groups we see **benefiting** from such permissive behavior are:

a) The pharmaceutical industry that sells the pills and devices, the doctors that prescribe them, the organizations that pretend to be the experts in sexual behavior for adolescents and obtain enormous grants to destroy the innocence of the young.

b) The mass media that tells teenagers that their sexual behavior can be gratified through rampant consumerism.

c) The multi-million dollar industry of pornography that encourages perverted sexual behavior that can end in addiction.

The ones that have **everything to lose** are:

a) Parents who lose their childrens' respect and society that is destroying its own roots and moral traditions.

b) The children that lose their innocence as they put their emotional, physical and psychological health at grave risk.

c) The taxpayers who have to pay for the irresponsible behavior of its adolescent population, especially through the increasing cost of health care directed towards teens and young adults.

People typically thrive on challenges set above them --like the pilot program in Lamar, Mo. where some 450 students tried the "pro-chastity" approach between 1987 and 1989. There were no pregnancies reported during that time. "Similar abstinence programs in 14 Midwestern schools are helping to change attitudes about premarital sex."

We are long overdue in recognizing once again that human beings, regardless of age, are distinguished from the animals in that we can control our own instincts. Teenagers are telling us through these statistics that they want to be challenged once more into controlling their instincts for the sake of their future. So let's once again bring back sanity, responsibility and leadership into our families, through programs encouraging abstinence, tradition and moral values.

CONCLUSIONS

1) Parents are the primary educators of their children in all matters, including human sexuality.

2) In providing an education in sexuality to their children, parents need to begin by denying the delusion that outside experts can do the job better than they can. Our program for parents is clear evidence of this. Since when have parents of the present generation been considered less capable of loving and educating their children in sexuality than their forebears? And why have they been so considered?

3) When others are permitted to serve as primary educators, parental authority is compromised and the parents' right and obligation to educate and protect their children is violated.

4) The excuse that because parents will not do it, the state has to intrude into the sensitive arena of sex education is nothing but an excuse to interfere with parental responsibility. This has resulted in the tragic consequences of plunging adolescents into premature promiscuous behavior with the accompanying results of:

   a) Increase in adolescent pregnancies
   b) Increase in venereal diseases
   c) Increased spread of AIDS
   d) Increase in suicides amongst adolescents
   e) Dramatic increase of abortions

STATISTICAL AND INFORMATIONAL SUMMARY

The following list is a summary of the findings in the field of problems with adolescent sexuality. It is broken down into the following categories:

a) THE GENERAL PROBLEM OF TEENAGE PROMISCUITY;

b) CONTRACEPTION AND TEENAGE PREGNANCY;

c) THE FAILURE OF CONTRACEPTIVE EDUCATION;

d) HEALTH RISKS OF ARTIFICIAL BIRTH CONTROL;

e) THE SOLUTION TO TEENAGE PROMISCUITY.

****

A. THE GENERAL PROBLEM OF TEENAGE PROMISCUITY

1. For more information, call (215) 424-7744 **The Parents' Coalition for Responsible Sex Education.**

2) Between 1960 and 1982, the number of live births per thousand for unmarried females aged 15 to 19 climbed from 15.3 to 28.9 (National Center for Health Statistics, 1980, 1984). ("The Role of Responsibility and Knowledge in Reducing Teenage Out-of-Wedlock Childbearing").

3) Based on recent polls by Lou Harris and by Grady Memorial Hospital, we get to the bottom line. 90% of teens admitted having become promiscuous simply because of peer pressure. 80% of sexual active teens say they were "drawn into it too soon." Only 14% of sexually active teens want clinics which provide contraceptives located in their schools. And finally, 84% of girls age 16 and under want their schools to teach them "how to say 'no' without hurting the person's feelings." (Quoted in Cal Thomas, Oct. 4, 1990; "Parents' Coalition for Responsible Sex Education", March 1991).

4. A study published in Pediatrics found that promiscuous girls were 2.5 times more likely to have used alcohol, 6.2 times more likely to have used marijuana, and 4.3 times more likely to have attempted suicide. Promiscuous boys were 2.8 times more likely to have used alcohol, 6.3 times more likely to have used marijuana, and 2.7 times more likely to have been in legal trouble. (**The Times-Picayune**, New Orleans, LA, 4/26/91).

5. Molly Kelly, author and lecturer, gave a talk in New Jersey, saying that: "chastity is not a profitable commodity to these organizations as are contraceptives and abortion, so therefore, it [chastity] is not encouraged." (Catholic Star Herald, Camden, NJ, 5/91).

B. CONTRACEPTION AND TEENAGE PREGNANCY

1) Planned Parenthood found a strong correlation between condom use and teenage pregnancy. Between 1976 and 1979, unmarried, sexually active women aged 15-19 who always used contraceptives had 19.2 percent increased pregnancies. During the same period, the pregnancy rate among women who had always used contraceptives rose 36.4 percent. (Josh McDowell, **The Myths of Sex Education**, p. 125).

2) The failure rate of condoms used by teenage girls to prevent pregnancy was 18.4% (**"Family Planning Perspectives,"** Vol. 18 [5]).

3) "Even among teens who use oral contraceptives regularly and follow the ideal pattern prescribed by Planned Parenthood, the pregnancy rate is 5.8 percent," (**"Family Planning "Perspectives**, Vol. 10 [3]).

4) The article from **The Parents' Coalition for Responsible Sex Education**, called "Now for a little condom sense," highlighted the following general findings:

   a. Condoms only offer limited protection, not Safe Sex.

   b. Sex education courses which discuss using contraceptives increase sexual activity.

   c. Pregnancy rates do not decrease (they may actually rise) as a result of distributing condoms.

   d. Both sexual activity and pregnancy rates decline when the value of delaying sexual activity is stressed.

5) The FDA has no performance standards for condoms. (Unpublished paper, Richard Smith, "The Condom, Oct. 1990, p.6)

6) "...one out of every five adolescents using condoms is pregnant at the end of a year." (Based on a failure rate of 18+ percent. William R. Grady et al., "Contraceptive Failure in the United States: Estimates from the 1962 National Survey of Family Growth," Family Planning Perspectives 18 no. 5 (1986): 207.

7) Quotes from "Now for a little condom sense:"

a. But a boy can only get a girl pregnant one week a month. An HIV positive partner can pass the virus 365 days a year.

b. All the "safe sex" message does is perpetuate risky behavior.

c. Faced with these results, sex educators are urging that contraceptives be distributed in the schools -- most often through a school-based clinic.

d. The January/February issue of Family Planning Perspectives further confirms the failure of this approach: a recent study of six urban school-based clinics shows that distributing contraceptives did not reduce the pregnancy rate and may have actually increased it.

C. THE FAILURE OF CONTRACEPTIVE EDUCATION

1) From 1970 to 1978, out-of-wedlock teenage births increased 79%. The birth rate among unmarried teens increased 81%. Abortions increased 180%. In the first eight years of the operation of Title X programs, the percentage of premarital pregnancies almost doubled. ("Clinics: cause or cure for teen pregnancy", May 1982).

2) "According to Dinah Richard, Ph.D., author of **Has Sex Education Failed Our Teenagers? A Research Report** (Pneuma Press), contraceptive education has failed, while abstinence education has proved effective. From 1971 to 1981, federal spending increased 306% for Family Planning; "there was a 48.3% increase in teen pregnancies and a 133% increase in abortions." (Condom Campaign Fails Miserably," Milwaukee Journal, Oct. 4, 1990).

3) In the 1980's, sex education programs expanded dramatically, with 80% of the States and nearly 90% of large public school districts requiring or encouraging sex education teaching. During this time period, pregnancy rates have risen. ("Data, Common Sense, and Teenage Pregnancy", Feb. 12, 1991).

4) Concerning distributing contraceptives in schools: "Researchers from Pediatrics, however, dismissed studies from the only clinics reporting success from such tactics as flawed." (James W. Stout and Frederick P. Rivera, "Schools and Sex Education: Does it Work? Pediatrics 83, #3 (1989) pg. 378).

5) Douglas Kirby, 'director of research of the Center for Population Options, an organization dedicated to sex education and school clinics,' in a 1988 report on the "Effectiveness of School Based-Clinics" said: "At the Center for Population Options, we have been engaging in a research project for several years on the impact of school-based clinics...We find basically that there are no measurable...I want to underline that word and put it in boldface..there is no measurable impact upon the use of birth control, nor upon pregnancy rates or birth rates." (Douglas Kirby, speaking at the Sixteenth Annual Meeting of the National Family Planning and Reproductive Health Association, 2 March 1988, Washington DC, as cited in Kasun).

6) 4% to 5% of students using six urban school-based clinics said they would have refrained from sexual intercourse if there had been no clinic in the school." (Douglas Kirby, et al. "Six School-Based Clinics: Their reproductive health Services and impact on Sexual Behavior," Family Planning Perspectives 23 no. 1 (1991) : 6-16).

7. The following quotes are from the article entitled "Condom campaigns fail miserably", the Milwaukee Journal, October 4, 1990:

a. The excuse given by those who promote condoms in schools and elsewhere is that too many young people are getting pregnant or infected with venereal diseases, and widely available condoms are the best way to combat both.

b. Dinah Richard's review of 33 sex education studies found that when contraceptive education was introduced there were gains in sexual knowledge, but shifts toward more liberal sexual attitudes, which led to promiscuity.

c. Dinah Richard describes one poll in which teens who have a sex education course that discusses contraceptives are shown to experience a 50% higher sexual activity rate than those who have taken a sex education course omitting contraceptives or who have not had any formal sex education.

D. HEALTH RISKS OF ARTIFICIAL BIRTH CONTROL

1. The International AIDS Conference of 1987 found that 30% of couples who knew their spouses were infected with AIDS and used condoms, caught the virus anyway; (Los Angeles Times, 8/10/88; A. Parachini, "AIDS-Condom Study Grant Cut Off by U.S.).

2. The 1987 Department of Health and Human Services report stated: "there are no clinical data supporting the value of condoms in preventing HIV; (Los Angeles Times, 8/18/87, A. Parachini, Condoms and AIDS: How Safe is Sex?).

3). Concerning the AIDS virus and the use of condoms,"the AIDS virus is 450 times smaller than the sperm." (American Journal of Nursing, vol. 87, #10, Nancy E. Dirubbo, "Condom Barrier;" 1987, pg. 1306).

4) Surgical gloves made of latex three times thicker than condoms have leaked blood. (Unpublished paper, Richard Smith, "The Condom, October 1990, pg. 13, and American Journal of Nursing, vol. 87, #10, Nancy E. Dirubbo, "Condom Barrier;" 1987, pg. 1306).

5) "Telling a person who engages in high-risk behavior to use a condom is like telling someone who is driving drunk to use a seatbelt. (U.S. Department of Education, "Will 'Safe Sex' Education Effectively Combat AIDS?", 22 January 1988, p. 16).

E. THE SOLUTION TO TEENAGE PROMISCUITY

1) In sharp contrast to "typical" school-based clinics, a program called Sexuality, Commitment, and Family, used by San Marcos Junior High, showed a decrease in pregnancy of 86% after two years of use. (Dinah Richard; Has Sex Education Failed Our Teenagers?, pg. 60)

2) The U.S. Department of Education is now calling for programs that teach the virtue of restraint, and use a moral context to present sexual education. To date the Federal Government has funded the development of over 100 such abstinence based curricula. (**U.S. Dept. of Education**, "AIDS and the Education of Our Children," Oct. 1987).

3) In Chicago, a curriculum called **Sex Respect** did a two-year follow up on their teens, who had 45% fewer pregnancies than non-participants (**Project Respect**, Box 87, Gulf, IL 60029).

4) In Atlanta, the Grady Memorial Hospital developed a curriculum that has been tested widely in that city's schools. Instead of concentrating on teaching kids how to use contraceptives, it instructs them on how and why to say "no" to sexual pressure. The results are astonishing: By the end of the eighth grade, students who had not taken the course were five times more likely to have become sexually active. (Marion Howard and Judith Blamey McCabe, "Helping Teenagers Postpone Sexual Involvement" Family Planning Perspectives 22 no 1 (1990) pg. 24).

5) Once a teen learns how to say "no" to teen sex, he can say "no" to other things as well. After implementing a program that encouraged abstinence and that taught study skills, the San Marcos school district in California reported better attendance, higher grades, higher test scores, and a drop in pregnancies from 147 to 20 [an 86% decrease]. (Teen Aid, Inc., N. 1330 Callspel, Spokane, WA 99201).

6) One abstinence pilot program at Lamar Junior High School in Lamar, Mo., was taught to about 450 students between 1987 and 1989. There were no pregnancies. School nurse Nancy Hughes attributes the success of the program to the values it teaches. Similar abstinence programs in 14 Midwestern schools helped change attitudes about premarital sex.

7) John Walsh, a spokesman for the Boston Archdiocese, was right when he said, "Our fear is that the state is sending the wrong message, 'Do whatever you want, but do it safely.' The state would be waging a campaign to encourage abstinence outside monogamous marital relationships, a campaign that says hedonism and promiscuity are not the way to go." The facts back him up. Condoms for children don't work. Abstinence programs do. Now it is up to parents to make sure the politicians get that message.

TITLE X QUOTES

Testimony of Charmaine Crouse Yoest; Policy Analyst, Family Research Council; Before the House of Representatives Committee on Energy and Commerce Subcommittee on Health and the Environment; March 19, 1991; The Reauthorization of Title X of the Public Health Service Act.

1. I would like to concentrate my comments on the efficiency of the portion of Title X that is allocated for services to adolescents. Although Title X provides family planning services to approximately 5 million women, many of them low-income, at least one-third of those reached are teenagers.

2. It is Title X's effect on teenagers that concerns us. The number of teenagers influences by this program is significant: an estimated 1.5 million teenagers are Title X clients, one-third of the program.

3. **FUNDING ISSUES:**

   a. Teenage births and abortions have increased at the same time Title X funding has increased.

   b. When Title X funding decreased, the numbers of increasing teen births and abortions leveled off. Between 1975 and 1980, as funding built up to its highest level, teen births increased 16%. Between 1980 and 1983, when funding was cut by $38 million (-23.5%), births increased only 3%. Then, between 1983 and 1987, funding increased by $18 million (14.5%) and births sped up again, increasing by 12.3%.

4. **DECLINING BIRTH RATES?**

   a. Title X advocates have long pointed to declining birth rates as evidence of their program's success. They fail, however, to delineate between marital and nonmarital teen births.

   b. Nonmarital teenage births have increased 61% over the life of Title X.

   c. A quarter of our nation's children are now born out-of-wedlock.

5. ACCOUNTABILITY

Title X is different from the other federal family planning programs in that it is targeted to service providers rather than individuals. Strangely, it has operated for twenty years with no accountability or measurement of effectiveness. There has never been an evaluation component included in the grants, and in 1983 the Department of Health and Human Services discontinued collecting client data. By pointing to declining birth rates Title X grantees have continued receiving more federal money. But in addition to using marital birth rates to get a drop in birth rates, leaving out the numbers of abortions has also been used as a way to show a statistical decline in births (implying pregnancies) and thereby to claim "success." It simply is not true: out-of-wedlock, unplanned pregnancies have risen drastically on Title X's watch.

Section Two: TEENAGE CONTRACEPTIVE USE AND MULTIPLE PARTNERS

MULTIPLE PARTNERS

According to the Centers for Disease Control: "The initiation of sexual intercourse early in life is associated with an increased number of sex partners and a greater risk for sexually transmitted diseases (STDs)." ("Premarital Sexual Experience Among Adolescent Women - United States, 1970-1988," Morbidity and Mortality Weekly Report, Centers for Disease Control, January 4, 1991, Volume 39, Nos. 51 & 52, p. 829).

There is evidence that contraceptive use leads to increased sexual activity, with a greater number of partners. (Cheryl D. Hayes, ed., **Risking the Future: Adolescent Sexuality, Pregnancy and Childbearing**, National Research Council, National Academy Press, Washington, DC 1987, p. 107.)

Family planning clinics, by dispensing prescription contraceptives without parental involvement, have exacerbated this trend. In fact, Dr. Robert Kistner of Harvard Medical School, and one of the developers of the oral contraceptive, now feels that use of contraceptives among teenagers is stimulating higher levels of promiscuity: "About ten years ago I declared that the pill would not lead to promiscuity. Well, I was wrong," he said. (**Family Practice News**, December 15, 1977, as quoted by James H. Ford and Michael Schwartz, "Birth Control for Teenagers: Diagram for Disaster," **Linacre Quarterly**, February 1979, p. 76).

45% of 15-24 year-olds who had initiated sexual intercourse before age 18 reported having had four or more partners; 75% reported having had two or more. (Morbidity and Mortality Weekly Report, p. 930).

Section Three: COMBATTING TEENAGE PREGNANCY WITH CONTRACEPTIVES

Jacqueline Darroch Forrest, Vice President of Research at the Alan Guttmacher Institute, was recently quoted in the Washington Post as saying: "The data are still saying that one-third of teens didn't use anything, not even the rhythm method." It seems that the intermediary goal of promoting contraceptive use has only been partially successful, nor has the ultimate objective of reducing unplanned pregnancies been achieved. Why? Because simply promoting contraceptive use is an ineffective, unrealistic and inappropriate means of combatting teenage pregnancy.

THE NATURE OF ADOLESCENT

Because of their developmental stage, adolescents are almost inevitably ineffective users of contraception. In Family Planning Perspectives, Marion Howard and Judith Blamey McCabe addressed this issue: "Until the age of 16, adolescents are still using concrete thinking skills. As a result, young teenagers have limited ability to recognize the potential impact of their choices; they are less likely than older teenagers to think about the future and to consider the consequences of their actions." (Marion Howard and Judith B. McCabe, "Helping Teenagers Postpone Sexual Involvement" Family Planning Perspectives, January/February 1990, Vol. 22, #1, p. 21).

Howard and McCabe go on to report that knowledge-based educational efforts with teenagers about sexuality and contraception do not result in increased contraceptive use. "The majority of young people in both the program and no-program groups who did have sex did not use contraceptives," they said. (They were not referring to a Title X program.)

INITIATION OF SEXUAL ACTIVITY

Research from Planned Parenthood shows that the number one reason, by far, that teenagers initiate sexual activity is peer pressure. By promoting contraceptive use among teenagers, we decrease the number of outside forces who are telling teenagers that it is okay not to have sex until marriage.

CONTRACEPTIVE FAILURE

The contraceptive approach to combatting unwed teenage pregnancy is flawed because of its high failure rate: one-third of teenage pregnancies occur while a contraceptive is being used. According to studies done by Professors John F. Katner and Melvin Zelnik of Johns Hopkins University, within one year of protected intercourse the pregnancy rate is 7.9%, within two years it is 13.6%. However, in actual use, 22.2% of sexually active contracepting teenagers become pregnant within one year and 34.8% within 2 years. (Scwartz, p. 146).

Section Four: SEXUALLY TRANSMITTED DISEASES

Discussions about teenage sexual activity too frequently focus on pregnancy as the only outcome to be avoided. In fact, teenagers involved in premarital sexual activity are threatened by a very high probability of contracting a sexually transmitted disease. According to the Center for Disease Control, adolescents have the highest risk of contracting an STD: 63% of STD's occur in the under 25 age bracket. By beginning sexual activity so early in their lives, their cumulative risk is staggering. If Title X clinics are indeed aiding and abetting unwed teenage sexual activity, as we believe they are, then they are contributing to a very disturbing societal trend. This is particularly troubling since a standard service offered at Title X clinics is screening for STDs:

- Since 1983 congenital syphilis has increased 15 times. Primary, secondary and early latent syphilis have increased 121% since 1985.

- Chlamydia has exploded - - 4 million cases recorded in 1990.

- An antibiotic-resistant gonorrhea has developed which has increased 50% yearly for the past five years.

Section Five: INFERTILITY

In addition to family planning services and screening for sexually transmitted diseases, Title X clinics also offer infertility counseling. Sexually transmitted diseases are a major contributor to infertility and other conception difficulties among women. Ectopic pregnancies, which can be caused by STDs, have quadrupled since 1970. It is a tragic irony that teenagers receiving family planning services from a Title X clinic may be returning later in life suffering from infertility as a result of STDs or abortion.

Section Six: THE OPTIMUM HEALTH MESSAGE

In a Washington Post editorial Eunice Kennedy Shriver has said:

"As a parent, I am not against the teaching of birth-control techniques to teenagers. But I, and parents like me, reject contraception as the first, best or only solution to the problem of teen pregnancy. To transform our schools into contraceptive dispensaries is to give a strong message that sex in adolescence is okay, that it is an approved extracurricular activity. 'Do what you please but do be careful' is the message we would be sending. Our society is obsessed with sex.

47-042 - 92 - 6

It is part of every message our teenagers receive - in their music, on television, in advertising, in the magazines they read, the role models they choose to emulate. But is sex to be thought of as just another appetite to be fed but not subject to inner controls? Adolescent needs will be fulfilled only when we begin to understand that teen-age pregnancy concerns the whole person, the family, the community and the society, not just the sexual act of the individual at risk." (Eunice Kennedy Shriver, "RX for Teen Pregnancy", The Washington Post, March 19, 1987.

Section Seven: TITLE X'S MANDATE

Title X's mandate is to reduce maternal and infant mortality and promote the health of mothers and children. The problems we have been describing in the program's approach to teenage pregnancy are preventing Title X from fulfilling this mandate. The continuing rise in teenage pregnancies contributes to our high rate of infant mortality, and sexually transmitted diseases negatively impact the health of both mothers and children.

INFANT MORTALITY

We have a national crisis in infant mortality -- America is 24th in the world in infant survival. One of the major causes of infant mortality is low birthweight, which is directly related to teenage pregnancy. The rate of infant mortality, and its reflection on the well-being of American children continues to be a national embarrassment at the same time that reducing infant mortality and promoting infant health have been major goals of Title X programming.

SEXUALLY TRANSMITTED DISEASES

STDs also hurt infants. The infection of infants from the mother's STDs has become a significant problem and will only continue increasing as nonmarital sexual activity remains unchecked.

Section Eight: EXECUTIVE ORDER 12606

The following questions must be asked of all federal programs:

a. Does the action by government strengthen or erode the stability of the family, and particularly, the marital commitment?

b. Does this action strengthen or erode the authority and rights of parents in the education, nurture, and supervision of their children?

c. Does this action help the family perform its functions, or does it substitute governmental activity for the function?

d. **What message does it send to young people concerning the relationship between their behavior, and their personal responsibility, and the norms of our society?**

By providing unemancipated, unwed minors with confidential (from their parents) family planning services, Title X clinics undermine the family in numerous ways:

1. **The authority and rights of parents are not only eroded, but completely undermined when sexual counseling and prescription contraceptives are dispensed without parental notification and involvement;**
2. **governmental activity is replacing an activity that is an integral family function; and**
3. **a message is sent to young people that premarital sexual activity is a norm of our society and that no permanent consequences will result from their behavioral choices. This message erodes the concept of marital commitment.**

FAMILY RESEARCH COUNCIL RECOMMENDATIONS

1. **Require a rigorous evaluation component in Title X.**
2. **Require substantial parental involvement if services to adolescents are continued.**
3. **Require Title X to promote postponement of sexual activity until marriage, and monogamy within marriage.**

(17)Family of the Americas Foundation (FAF) is a non-profit

PREPARED STATEMENT OF ROBERT WM. BLUM, M.D., PH.D., PROFESSOR AND DIRECTOR, DIVISION, GENERAL PEDIATRICS & ADOLESCENT HEALTH, UNIVERSITY OF MINNESOTA, MINNEAPOLIS, MN

I am Dr. Robert Blum, Professor in Pediatrics and the Director of the Division of General Pediatrics and Adolescent Health at the University of Minnesota. I am also the President of the Society for Adolescent Medicine, the largest professional organization in the United States, with over 1100 health care professionals dedicated to adolescent health.

I do not need to tell this committee of the problems facing youth today, but I do need to say that the problems are widespread. The problems facing youth are not isolated to the inner cities and reservation communities of America, but are in Scarsdale, Evanston and La Jolla as well. To give you a sense of the scope of the issues, in 1987 we surveyed over 36,000 7-12th graders in Minnesota--all children were in school and there was an equal distribution of those from economically impoverished as well as from economically advantaged homes. The sample was urban and rural. What did we find?

- By the 12th grade 70% of urban teens and 55% of rural teens had had intercourse. There is almost no difference between males and females. There is almost no difference based on religion.

- 6% of the population report having intercourse by the age of 10. The majority of those did not consider it abuse.

- The average age for intercourse was approximately 13.5 years for males and 14.5 years for females.

- Nearly 15% of girls report having been sexually abused; a slightly smaller percent report physical abuse.

- Large numbers of teens are at high risk for suicide.

- More than one in five 12th-grade urban females report having attempted to kill themselves at least once.

- More than 10% of urban high school students qualify by their responses as being under extreme stress.

- High suicide risk varies dramatically by ethnicity. For example, for urban high school females, the following are percents at high risk for suicide:
  - White 7.9%
  - African-American 9.0%
  - Hispanic 16.7%
  - Native American 14.8%
  - Asian 19.5%

I could go on and on, but there is no need. The data are clear -- these are your children and mine; and these are your grandchildren.

What do we know that makes a difference in the lives of teens, especially those who are disadvantaged due to poverty?

- We know that the following factors put teens at risk:
  - poverty
  - parental unemployment
  - parental substance use

- physical/sexual abuse

- We know that those who have emotional support from an adult do better than peers who do not. While preferable for the adult to be a parent, it is not fundamental for resiliency.
- Where there is a community (e.g., school, church) that recognizes and rewards competencies and determination, children do better.
- Resilient teens tend to grow up in families which have been able to access family planning services and thereby limit family size.
- School-based interventions (e.g., education, mentoring, counselling, health services) improve the outcomes for teenagers at risk.

What should be the role of the federal government regarding high risk youth? First, there needs to be a willingness to invest in education of our children. At present there appears to be no will to address this central issue at either the federal or state levels despite the fact that we know there is an inverse correlation at the state level between educational investment and the number of prison cells. There is need for a federally led initiative in education.

Secondly, the federal government should encourage new initiatives for those young people (nearly half our population) who are vocationally rather than academically oriented. Other than college, our post-secondary school options are weak.

Third, federal agencies should move from primarily supporting demonstration grants with the goal of developing new interventions to supporting dissemination and replication programs of those interventions which have been shown to be effective. We spend a lot of time demonstrating what we already know; and there are few resources available to adapt and apply interventions of proven efficacy.

Fourth, the federal bureaucracy is currently set up to address issues on a categorical basis; thus, it is rarely feasible to develop cross-cutting interventions (e.g., interventions which address school failure, pregnancy risk and substance abuse concurrently), despite the fact that we know that many high risk behaviors are interrelated. Congress should encourage and mandate more interagency collaboration and pooling of resources.

Fifth, over the past decade it has become increasingly clear that the central problems of high risk youth are not amenable to change through the two-year demonstration project. Whether it is "self-esteem building" classes or "Just say No" classes these limited interventions work for only a very narrow band of the teen population. For those most "at risk", the problems are complex and rarely amenable to simple interventions. Increasingly, foundations have become aware of this and, as a consequence, the private sector is choosing to invest its limited resources in groups of "at risk" children with a commitment of maintaining support for 15-20 years. Eugene Lange, in New York, showed that real and ongoing support makes a difference in the lives of kids. The federal government is handicapped by an electoral process every two years which creates a political disincentive for doing the very thing we know would make a difference.

Finally, to be effective, Congress on both sides of the aisle--political conservatives and liberals alike--would be well advised to lay aside their support for interventions which reflect little else beyond their religious or social biases and rather take a hard look at 15 years of intervention programs in America. Were Congress to do so, one would find many programs that work and are worth supporting and expanding. One would also find hundreds of millions of dollars wasted on programs which were ill-conceived and garnered support only because they reflected the biases of those in the majority at that time.

And one would see in the horizon opportunity, not despair-opportunity to improve the health and social functioning among those youths who are most at risk in our society for bad things happening to them.

Thank you for the opportunity to share with you my perspective on where we are and what we could be doing to improve the outcomes for high risk youth in America.

11M07LB490

PREPARED STATEMENT OF BRIAN L. WILCOX, PH.D., DIRECTOR, LEGISLATIVE AFFAIRS AND POLICY STUDIES, WASHINGTON, DC

American Psychological Association

Advancing psychology as a science, a profession, and as a means of promoting human welfare

July 2, 1991

The Honorable Patricia Schroeder
Chairwoman
Select Committee on Children, Youth and Families
385 Annex II
Washington, DC 20515

Dear Representative Schroeder:

I am writing on behalf of the membership of the American Psychological Association to thank you for holding hearings recently on "The Risky Business of Adolescence." The hearings produced several thoughtful analyses of the issue of risk-taking behaviors of adolescents as well as some interesting proposals for action. Given the life-threatening consequences of several forms of risk-taking, it is our hope that Congress will search for ways to seriously address this set of problems.

Having had an opportunity to review the testimony presented, I would like to comment on the testimony provided by Kathleen M. Sullivan regarding Project Respect. I believe this testimony was extremely misleading and contained several factual errors which should not go unchallenged.

Project Respect has been supported in part by funds authorized by the Adolescent Family Life Act and administered through the Office of Adolescent Pregnancy Programs (OAPP) in the Department of Health and Human Services. OAPP supported an evaluation of the program operated by Project Respect, known as "Sex Respect." My comments will make reference to both the claims made in Ms. Sullivan's testimony and the conclusions drawn by the evaluation report submitted to OAPP by the evaluation team.

When Ms. Sullivan speaks of the success of the program, she refers to only one general type of outcome measures--attitudinal change. The problem with an exclusive focus on changing attitudes is that the relationship between attitudes and behavior is often surprisingly weak. Indeed, Ms. Sullivan failed to mention that the one question focusing on the behavior of participants in the Sex Respect program found no effect for the program, though I'll say more about this later. One likely explanation for significant changes in attitude measures in the absence of behavioral change is that the attitude change is ephemeral, reflecting nothing more than the respondents wanting to provide a "socially desirable" response.

It is quite customary in evaluation research to independently measure the propensity of the respondents to answer questions in a socially desirable manner. The evaluators of the Sex Respect program failed to do so and thus are unable to rule out this competing explanation for the results.

It should also be noted that not all of the results are as robust as Ms. Sullivan's testimony suggests. For example, though the program has a goal of increasing communication between teen and parent regarding matters of sexuality and sexual behavior, only a minority of the participants report that they discussed the course material with their parents. Another problem in interpreting the results stems from the evaluators' use of inappropriate statistical techniques which result in a higher likelihood of drawing false inferences.

The "bottom line" goal of Sex Respect is to encourage sexual abstinence. Changing attitudes but not behavior will not reduce adolescent pregnancy or sexually transmitted disease rates. The evaluation of Sex Respect indicates very clearly that, in this regard, the program failed to achieve its main objective. Students who were participants in the Sex Respect program were no less sexually active after 12 and 24 months than were a roughly comparable group of students who had not participated in the program. The evaluators provided no data regarding other important behavioral outcomes (e.g., pregnancy rates, abortion rates, incidence of sexually transmitted diseases, etc.).

This information, drawn from an evaluation conducted by researchers sympathetic to the aims of Sex Respect, clearly suggests that Ms. Sullivan's enthusiasm for and endorsement of the program and her advocacy for its expansion are not warranted. Contrary to Ms. Sullivan's claim in her testimony, the program has demonstrated neither its effectiveness nor its cost effectiveness.

Abstinence education should be a part of any sex education curriculum. Many adolescents wish to abstain from sexual activity, for a variety of reasons, and need assistance in developing the cognitive and behavioral strategies for doing so. Other adolescents, though, will become sexually active despite any and all encouragement to the contrary. These adolescents must be given the knowledge and skills they will need to both protect and promote their physical and emotional health. Programs focusing exclusively on abstinence, though well intentioned, may actually place many teens at greater risk for pregnancy, disease, and emotional trauma. Adults, including policymakers, who fail to understand these "facts of life" do a disservice to us all.

Again, thank you for your leadership in addressing these important issues. Please feel free to call upon me if the American Psychological Association can be of further assistance.

Sincerely,

Brian L. Wilcox, Ph.D.
Director,
Legislative Affairs and
Policy Studies

PREPARED STATEMENT OF DAMON K. MARQUIS, DIRECTOR OF HEALTH EDUCATION, NATIONAL COMMISSION ON CORRECTIONAL HEALTH CARE, CHICAGO, IL

Thank you for the opportunity to present information to you on behalf of the National Commission on Correctional Health Care (NCCHC) focusing on the health issues facing our nation's youth passing through the juvenile justice system. My name is Damon K. Marquis and I am currently the Director of Health Education for NCCHC.

NCCHC offers the only national juvenile health education training program for incarcerated youth. We have pioneered the effort to provide comprehensive health education for this high risk population. The program actively and successfully promotes education and behavior change for youth who practice high risk behavior. It is funded in part through a cooperative agreement with the Centers for Disease Control.

There are approximately 600,000 youth admitted to public juvenile facilities annually. On any given day, over 55,000 youth are held in public facilities. Sixty percent of the youth in public facilities are youth of color.

According to the Office of Juvenile Justice and Delinquency Prevention report on Children in Custody in 1989, eleven percent of all juveniles in public facilities were held for drug related offenses. Forty nine percent of these were held for distribution. The total number of juveniles held for alcohol or other drug offenses increased 150 percent from 1985 to 1989.

In an attempt to gain further information on the health of incarcerated youth, NCCHC has implemented a limited Youth Risk Behavior Survey (YRBS) in our nation's juvenile facilities. Questions on the survey address various health issues including alcohol and other substance use, sexual behavior, violence and suicide. The survey is being conducted in five states, including: Massachusetts, New York, Tennessee, Texas, and Wisconsin.

Although only a portion of the survey results are in, preliminary results give us some very useful information. Of the responses received to date, approximately 90% of the youth had tried cigarette smoking, almost 80% of these having done so before the age of 15. Less than 9% of respondents report never drinking alcohol in his/her life while nearly 35% report having at least one drink of alcohol 100 or more days in their life. Eighty-one percent of the youth surveyed to date have reported trying marijuana while 32% reported trying cocaine in some form. Nine percent of the respondents have reported injecting drugs.

The survey results thus far suggest that over 90% of the youth responding have been sexually active. Fifty-six percent of these youth report not using a condom the last time they willingly had sex (i.e. were not forced to have sex). In response to the question addressing sexual abuse, 17% have reported being abused. Youth are also asked if they have ever been or gotten someone pregnant and 27% report at least one occurrence; 13% report two or more occurrences.

In responding to questions on suicide, 31% of the respondents have reported seriously considering attempting suicide and 27% report actually making a suicide plan. Twenty-one percent report actually attempting suicide at least once in the past 12 months, nearly 16% of these report attempting suicide six or more times.

As I have stated, this data is based on initial data received from a survey limited to randomly selected juvenile facilities in five states. These statistics are likely to change as more data are received. Additionally, these results can not be generalized to all youth in juvenile facilities nationwide. To do this would require a much more extensive research program. A final report on this project will be available in the fall of 1991.

The information from the current survey does suggest some very important trends in behavior that must be addressed when working with these youth. NCCHC's youth training program is offered throughout the country to staff working directly with youth in these facilities. Participants learn the latest information regarding HIV infection and AIDS, sexually transmitted diseases (STDs), and substance use. The program is also actively working to incorporate information on teen parenting and violence. The goal of this program is to give staff working with youth the necessary tools to intercede in high risk behavior and attitudes. The training program focuses on identifying health risk behavior, assessing the risk with the youth and providing appropriate intervention and referral. Particular focus is placed on behaviors placing the youth at greater risk for HIV infection.

Trainers providing this program report that juvenile staff attending the training are enthusiastic about the information they obtain. Depending on the length of stay of the youth, the time during which a youth is incarcerated is an excellent time to provide education and intervention. The challenge to the staff working with the youth is to provide all of the necessary information in the time allotted <u>and</u> help the youth see that making behavior changes that are life enhancing will benefit him\her in the future. For many of these youth, planning for the future is a difficult concept when surviving the next 24 hours has been their only experience to date.

For those youth prepared to begin to make behavior changes while in juvenile facilities, staff must be prepared to assist in the continuation of care after the youth leaves the facility. NCCHC encourages staff attending its training to network with community based organizations. Participants are provided with a variety of resources as an initial boost to their networking effort. The intent is for staff in juvenile facilities to work with staff from community based organizations to assure after-care for the youth.

In conclusion, I would like to stress the importance of comprehensive health education to incarcerated youth. Many of these youth have not received the benefit of conventional health educational resources because they were out of school and/or homeless and/or runaways prior to being placed in juvenile facilities. For others, this may be the only time a proactive, health education program is offered in any setting. This is an excellent opportunity to provide the youth with the information and resources necessary to make vital behavior changes.

In order to accomplish this, monies must be made available to enhance the educational opportunities of staff and residents in juvenile facilities. Networks between juvenile facilities and community based organizations must be encouraged and fostered. Most importantly, we must be prepared as a society to accept these youth as vital, important and productive future citizens--not delinquents who we have forgotten. We must reach out to them where they are in their lives emotionally, psychologically and developmentally. We must be prepared to stand up for these youth and show them that they can make a difference in our society.

It is the National Commission's belief that substantial inroads can be made in health education and behavior change for youth. For this reason, NCCHC is committed to its Health Education Training for Incarcerated Youth and to providing this program to as many youth workers as is possible.

I appreciate this opportunity to present this information to you. If NCCHC can provide members of the Committee or the general public with any further information, we would be pleased to be of assistance. NCCHC is located at 2105 N. Southport, Suite 200, Chicago, IL 60614. Our phone number is (312) 528-0818.

Thank you.

Prepared Statement of Janet Shalwitz, M.D., Director, Special Programs for Youth, San Francisco, CA

Special Programs for Youth, a division of the San Francisco Department of Public Health provides comprehensive health care services to youth who are homeless, runaway, and involved in the juvenile justice system. Primary care clinics are housed in 2 community based agencies which serve as the focal points for activities/services re homeless and runaway youth; the juvenile detention facility; the juvenile probation department; and a long term facility for serious male offenders. Each year over 4,500 youth are seen. These youth represent the highest risk (for HIV, pregnancy, STDs, school drop-out, homicide, etc.) youth in San Francisco. The youth are 60% male; 46% African American, 18% Latino, 26% White, 8% Asian/PI, and 2% other; 11 - 23 years with a mean age of 16. Unlinked HIV Seroprevalence studies conducted in the Special Programs for Youth Primary Care Clinics reveal almost 4% of this population (sample size of 784) and 5% of the males (n=465) are infected with HIV. Of the 19 males who self identify as engaging in male homosexual/bisexual behaviors and intravenous drug use over 50% are HIV+. Males who engage in homosexual/bisexual behaviors without intravenous drug use (n=30) have a seroprevalence rate of 30%.

Prevention activities with youth vary depending on the specific needs and risks of the individual clients as well as the setting of the services. Regardless of where youth are seen, STDs, HIV, and pregnancy are highly visible issues which are thoroughly integrated into all aspects of primary care including street outreach, triage, screening, episodic and comprehensive visits. All youth are assessed for risky behaviors, provided with risk reduction counseling, offered HIV confidential counseling and testing, as well as provided with comprehensive primary care. Additionally, partners are encouraged to come to medical visits together in order to discuss negotiating and practicing safe sex. All youth are offered free condoms and bleach.

It is well recognized this work alone will not have an impact on changing behaviors of high risk youth. For most youth HIV is not a high priority. The youth are concerned with food, shelter, friends, family, recreation, school, money, safety, etc. They live in a variety of cultures and communities which do not have a homogeneous nor necessarily a concerned view re HIV.

Our work is just one piece of the prevention efforts targetting high risk youth. Health care providers work in concert with the youth service agencies which address their multiple other needs including housing, recreation, job readiness and training, group work (support, youth and family counseling, 12 step programs, etc.) and case management. These collective prevention efforts take place wherever youth can be reached including abandoned buildings, parks, streets, shelters, multiservice and counseling centers, schools, the detention facility, as well as clinics. Prevention messages and activities are included within the context of all these services and are regularly reinforced. Free condom and bleach distribution is widespread.

Recommendations:

1) Vigorous targetted prevention efforts should be undertaken focusing on youth who are highest risk for HIV which must specifically include sexual minority (gay, bisexual, lesbian, transvestite, transsexual) youth .

2) Prevention efforts which have a goal of behavior change require a community-wide multiagency collaborative approach in order to integrate HIV prevention messages into the daily and routine culture of the community. This process requires a long term plan and commitment.

3) Primary care services specially designed for youth should be located where large numbers of youth congregate. These services should work in cooperation with other youth serving agencies in order to optimize staff skills and provide prompt and appropriate referrals for youth with multiple needs. HIV confidential counseling and testing should be included in the provision of comprehensive primary care. Every staffperson in the primary care team must be specially trained to effectively perform this work.

4) Training and education for all staff who work with youth must be ongoing and tailored for the specific needs and responsibilities of the staff. Knowledge about HIV must be integrated into the everyday experiences which bring a person into contact with a young person.

5) HIV infected youth and their loved ones must be included in the planning, design, implementation, and evaluation of these prevention efforts.

Prepared Statement of American Academy of Pediatrics, Washington, DC

The American Academy of Pediatrics, on behalf of its 41,000 Fellows who are dedicated to the promotion of infant, child and adolescent health, appreciates the opportunity to submit these formal comments on "The Risky Business of Adolescence: How to Help Teens Stay Safe." We also wish to applaud the Committee, and particularly the distinguished chairwoman, for focusing overdue public attention on vulnerable--and still struggling--American youth.

The consequences of adolescent risk-taking behavior cannot be overstated. Teenagers and young adults represent the only segment of the United States population for whom mortality has risen over the past quarter century. Not only do such lamentable data compare unfavorably with rates for children and adults, but they also demonstrate that our country lags far behind our peers in Europe and elsewhere with respect to these all-important measurements of social progress.

The rate of adolescent mortality in America is the highest in the industrialized world. The three leading causes of death within this age group--injury, homicide and suicide--are all behavioral in origin.

There is also, of course, extensive morbidity among American youth. Consequences of developing sexuality include more than one million adolescent pregnancies annually, roughly 250,000 reported cases of sexually transmitted diseases, and a soaring rate of HIV infection. Here too, despite evidence that our rate of adolescent sexual activity parallels that of comparable nations, the rate of pregnancy in the U.S. "leads" the industrialized world.

More than 90 percent of our high school seniors have tried alcohol, with two-thirds drinking at least once per month. Fully 20 percent of our high school seniors are regular users of marijuana, with approximately 5 percent drinking alcohol or smoking marijuana daily. Rates among school dropouts are even higher.

Nearly 5000 adolescents and young adults die annually from suicide--more than 500,000 survive such attempts, if only physically. Approximately 1 million American teenagers have a diagnosable chronic illness or disabling condition.

The causes of our excess mortality and morbidity are multiple, and interestingly they relate to issues both of access and lack of access. Broad access to drugs, automobiles, guns, and a social environment (including the media) which often promotes risk-taking behavior, contributes mightily to our alarming rate of serious health consequences. By contrast, obstacles to access to health services prevent many teenagers from receiving the care and counseling which might positively impact on their behaviors and dysfunctions.

These obstacles are both financial and geographic. Within the United States adolescents are likelier than is any other age group to be uninsured or under-insured for health care services. One of every seven adolescents, and one of every three adolescents below the poverty level, have no health insurance. Even when insured, adolescents' coverage most frequently does not include preventive care, counseling or substance abuse treatment. These financial constraints invariably force the adolescent to rely solely on episodic care for acute illness. This type of care addresses none of the issues which are of deepest concern in our attempts to alter profound risk-taking behavior (with its attendant mortality and morbidity).

Even if finances were not an issue, regional deficiencies in the availability of health care to adolescents would remain an obstacle to our best efforts to reduce risk-taking behavior. Ideally, every adolescent should have a "medical home" where care could be provided in a continuous and comprehensive fashion. A personal physician with a knowledge of the young person over time, as well as with a strong relationship with parents and other family members, remains the most promising means of providing the care and guidance which are indispensable to securing safer behavior in young persons.

Unfortunately, in many areas of our country, both urban and rural, this model of care is still unavailable. It is beyond debate that (in these special circumstances of physician scarcity) alternatives should be developed to fill the vacuum. Among such alternatives would certainly be school-based health care, which seeks to provide an impressive complement of services (logically) within the environment in which the adolescent is to be found. Beyond acute episodic care, these school-based services should be prepared to offer the evaluation and counseling essential to prevent (or in any case address) risk-taking behavior. Such services should be used to promote abstinence from drug use and sexual activity; to provide counseling for those who choose to be sexually active; to recognize the early signs of mental illness, including depression, suicidal tendencies and potential violence; and to assure treatment, either on site or by referral, of those conditions which place a young person at continuing peril.

As risk-taking behavior among adolescents is of urgent (or at least substantially growing) concern throughout the nation, and since the causes of such behavior are multiple, our interventions as advocates for children and youth must be imaginative, comprehensive and not limited to any single model or methodology. Regrettably, we cannot expect all vulnerable adolescents to come to our offices for care. The times require us now to pursue aggressively the full range of alternatives necessary to provide adolescents with access to desperately needed health services. Under the forceful new leadership of this Committee, the Academy pledges its unswerving commitment to that end.

PREPARED STATEMENT OF MARK PAUL LEHMAN, HUMAN RIGHTS CAMPAIGN FUND, WASHINGTON, DC

SUMMARY

America's youth are this nation's greatest resource. Unfortunately, we are neglecting to provide our youth with sufficient information, education, social skills, and support they need to remain healthy and in school.

Adolescents need to receive more health prevention education in order to reduce the number of unwanted pregnancies, transmission of HIV disease, and suicide.

Lesbian and gay youth are a population that has been particularly neglected. These youth are two to three times more likely to attempt suicide and are at great risk for HIV and STDs.

There is a growing recognition among educators and child welfare advocates that services that attempt to reach out to youth at risk -- including lesbian and gay youth -- save lives and keep adolescents in school, off the streets, and healthy.

YOUTH AT RISK FOR HIV

American youth are at great risk of contracting HIV disease and our current efforts to reduce this risk among adolescents are failing. These youth lack the information, the social skills, and the support they need to protect themselves.

The Centers for Disease Control reported that more than 20 percent of all persons with AIDS are 20 to 29 years of age. Given the long latency period between infection and the onset of the disease, many were likely infected as adolescents.

While those statistics are alarming, even more alarming is the increase of adolescents with AIDS -- over the past two years, the number of adolescents with AIDS increased from 325 to 675. The Center for Population Options reports that each year, one in six teen-agers contracts a sexually transmitted disease.

Gay and lesbian youth, a population at great risk of HIV infection, have been frequently ignored in efforts to reduce the spread of AIDS among adolescents. A 1990 study by the General Accounting Office found that "homosexual youth, particularly males, are of specific concern as they have been one of the high-risk groups for HIV transmission in the United States. As youth, these teens also search for their identity and struggle to establish satisfying relationships, leading them, in some cases, to experiment with heterosexual affiliations. This places lesbian youth, who generally would be in a low-risk category, at heightened risk of infection. Such exploration also serves as a possible link between heterosexual and homosexual youth in the transmission of

HIV." (AIDS Education, Public School Programs Require More Student Information and Teacher Training, GAO/HRD-90-103)

AIDS education programs are not widely available in health clinics, community centers, or schools -- and many AIDS education programs that currently exist do not address the needs specific to lesbian and gay youth.

LESBIANS AT RISK FOR TEEN PREGNANCY

Because many gay and lesbian youth experiment with heterosexual affiliations (as cited above from the 1990 AIDS Education GAO study), lesbian youth are at a high risk for unintentional pregnancy. Health clinics, community services, and schools need to address the needs specific to lesbian and gay youth in order to reduce this risk.

LESBIAN AND GAY YOUTH

Many adolescents identify themselves as lesbian or gay, or engage in same-sex sexual activity. Unfortunately, these youth face prejudice and discrimination at a crucial developmental stage in their lives. Such prejudice and discrimination frequently leads to harassment, ostracism, and even violence against them. Many schools and health clinics have not provided the support these youth need to develop a strong self-esteem.

Because lesbian and gay youth face rejection and abuse both at home and school, these youth are at great risk for a variety of psychosocial problems and self-destructive behavior such as school failure, substance abuse, unwanted pregnancy, and suicide. These youth are likely to run away from home and drop out of school. While some of these youth may enter the child welfare system, without special social services targeted to reach these youth, many will remain outside any system of care. Lesbian and gay youth who are fortunate enough to enter the child welfare system, frequently find this system unsympathetic to their needs.

According to the Report of the Secretary's Task Force on Youth Suicide (HHS, 1989) and a recent study in the Journal of the American Academy of Pediatrics (June 1991), gay and lesbian youth are two to three times more likely to attempt suicide than their heterosexual peers.

The HHS Report noted that "many suicidal youth tend to be lonely, isolated, and withdrawn with few social support systems. For many, traditional family structure no longer exists. Gay youth face rejection and abuse from family members and are often unwelcome in youth groups or recreational activities. For whatever reasons, some youth avoid or are systematically excluded from group activities. Efforts to integrate these high risk young people into the mainstream may ameliorate the risk of suicide. Specialized groups may be required to fulfill specific needs for some groups of young people."

PROGRAMS THAT ARE HELPING LESBIAN AND GAY YOUTH

Many adolescents identify themselves as lesbian or gay, or engage in same-sex sexual activity. Unfortunately, these youth face prejudice and discrimination at a crucial developmental stage in their lives. Such prejudice and discrimination frequently leads to harassment, ostracism, and even violence against them. Unfortunately, many schools and health clinics have not provided the support these youth need.

Because lesbian and gay youth face rejection and abuse both at home and school, these youth are at great risk for a variety of psychosocial problems and self-destructive behavior such as school failure, substance abuse, unwanted pregnancy, and suicide. These youth are likely to run away from home and drop out of school. While some of these youth may enter the child welfare system, without special social services targeted to reach these youth, many will remain outside any system of care. Lesbian and gay youth who enter the child welfare system, frequently find this system unsympathetic to their needs.

School districts and communities that provide services and education that take into account the needs of lesbian and gay youth are working to save lives and keep youth healthy, at home, and in school.

Recognizing the difficulties that lesbian and gay youth face, the National Education Association passed a resolution in 1989 that stated: "All persons, regardless of sexual orientation, should be afforded equal opportunity within the public education system. The Association further believes that every school district should provide counseling for students who are struggling with their sexual/gender orientation."

In 1985-86, the Los Angeles Unified School District developed "Project 10" -- a model program of services for students who self-identify as gay or lesbian or students who express conflicts over their sexual orientation. Originally begun as a drop-out prevention program, Project 10 evolved into general counseling and education vehicle for both the gay and non-gay school population. The Project 10 model provides for education, school safety, drop-out prevention strategies, and support services. Other school districts in California have developed programs modeled after Project 10.

Several other communities have developed programs that attempt to reach homeless gay and lesbian youth, to get them off the street, and when possible, to return to school and their families.

FAILED ATTEMPTS TO CURTAIL EFFORTS TO HELP LESBIAN AND GAY YOUTH

In the past three years, a few Members of Congress have attempted to restrict local school programs that reach out to lesbian and gay youth by restricting funding to schools in the Labor, HHS, and Education Appropriations bill. These attempts failed.

In 1988 and 1989, the Senate adopted an amendment proposed by Senator Gordon Humphrey stating that "None of the funds made available by this Act, shall be used to produce or distribute materials directed at the teaching of school children and which promote or encourage homosexuality or use words stating that homosexuality is 'normal,' 'natural,' or 'healthy.'"

In both years, the House-Senate conference deleted the Humphrey amendment but retained a Cranston amendment stating: "AIDS education programs that receive assistance from the Centers for Disease Control and other education curricula dealing with sexual activity that receive assistance under this Act, (1) shall not be designed to promote or encourage, directly, intravenous drug abuse or sexual activity, homosexual or heterosexual; and (2) with regards to AIDS education programs and curricula, (A) shall be designed to reduce exposure to and transmission of the etiologic agent for acquired immune deficiency syndrome by providing accurate information; and (B) shall provide information on the health risks of promiscuous sexual activity and intravenous drug abuse."

Everyone agrees that it is not the role of the government to encourage sexual activity -- heterosexual or homosexual. This is what Congress decreed, in the 1989 Cranston amendment, for all federal education programs dealing with sexuality.

Restrictions like the Humphrey amendment remove the right of each school district, in consultation with teachers, counselors, and parents, to choose the curriculum and materials most appropriate for its students according to the standards of the local community.

Given the high rate of gay youth suicide, runaway gay youth, and the spread of AIDS in the adolescent population, federal restrictions would limit the ability of educators, counselors, and health officials to deal effectively with the attitudes underlying these problems.

RECOMMENDATIONS TO HELP TEENS STAY SAFE

* **Adolescents need access to persistent comprehensive health care that includes health prevention education.**

Many children fail to receive adequate health care either through the child welfare system or the community. School health clinics can encourage health prevention education.

A recent survey by the Roper Organization found that an overwhelming majority of Americans believe that children as young as 12 should receive information about AIDS from their schools (Washington Post, June 26, 1991).

Pregnancy, HIV and other sexually transmitted diseases, and drug abuse prevention education should begin at an early age and should continue throughout an adolescent's school years. Education should be frank and include information on prevention of HIV transmission.

School districts should not rely on one-shot intense educational effort to combat these enormous problems.

* **Prevention programs for HIV transmission -- and other risky behaviors such as drug abuse -- must be judged by increased knowledge, changes in attitudes and inducement of actual behavioral changes.**

While the majority of Americans understand that sexual abstinence is an effective way for a youth to remain HIV-negative, only one in seven believe that abstinence is a realistic solution to HIV transmission. The statistics show that our youth are becoming sexually active at an early age. We must provide them with adequate information and support so that they are able to make healthy and responsible decisions about sexual activity.

AIDS education messages should be innovative and diverse, using many channels to communicate this message.

We cannot be satisfied with adolescent AIDS education efforts until sufficient research shows that those efforts are leading to behavioral changes among adolescents.

* **The Public Health Service should conduct a comprehensive study on the sexual behavior of adolescents.**

A key component to produce AIDS prevention education efforts that create behavioral changes among adolescents is adequate information about the sexual behavior of youth.

* **Adolescents should have access to condoms through school health clinics and various community organizations.**

Again according to a recent Roper Organization survey, 47 percent of the American public support condom distribute in junior high schools.

This shows the growing understanding that because we cannot deny that adolescents have and continue to engage in sexual activity, adolescents must have access to condoms and be taught to protect themselves with the use of condoms.

* **Health prevention education needs to be targeted specifically to lesbian and gay youth.**

We can no longer ignore this population of adolescents. Educational programs need to be certain that their information and messages of prevention reach these youth and are specific to their needs.

* **The Department of Health and Human Services should encourage school districts and communities to fully implement the recommendations of the Secretary's Task Force on Youth Suicide.**

Many of America's youth are at great risk for suicide. Gay and lesbian youth are among the largest populations that attempt suicide. Implementation of these recommendations would be a first step in addressing this American tragedy.

* **Given the difficulties facing lesbian and gay youth, more research is needed to identify and serve the needs of this population at risk.**

PREPARED STATEMENT OF THE CENTER FOR POPULATION OPTIONS, WASHINGTON, DC

The Center for Population Options (CPO) is a nonprofit educational organization dedicated to improving the quality of life for adolescents by preventing unintended teenage pregnancy and too-early childbearing. Through its domestic and international programs, CPO seeks to improve adolescent decision-making through "life planning" and other educational programs, to improve access to reproductive and basic health care, and to prevent the spread among adolescents of HIV and other sexually transmitted diseases.

For the first time in almost two decades, the birth rate among teenagers in the United States is rising. In 1988, 488,961 teenagers gave birth, accounting for 12.5 percent of all births. Almost one-quarter of these births were to adolescents who already had one or more children. The increase in birth rates was sharpest among young teens, ages 15 to 17 - 10% in the span of two years. The United States has the highest teen pregnancy rate of all developed countries, almost twice that of England, France and Canada, and more than six times that of the Netherlands. More than a million girls become pregnant in this country every year; almost half of them give birth. For policy-makers and the public, these numbers are dismaying. For the hundreds of thousands of teenage girls becoming mothers too soon, they are devastating.

Because numerous factors contribute to the epidemic rates of teen pregnancy and sexually transmitted diseases among adolescents, no single approach to solving these problems can hope to succeed. However, lack of access to health information and services for adolescents clearly contributes to the present crises. CPO is committed to a comprehensive approach to adolescent health care that addresses both the risk and the risk-taking behavior and includes health education, access to services, self-esteem and skills-building.

Through the Support Center for School-Based Clinics, CPO provides information, training and technical assistance to communities seeking to meet the unique health needs of adolescents and facilitate access to critical services by establishing a health facility on or near school grounds.

Since the first school-based clinic (SBC) was founded in 1970, the concept has gained enthusiastic support from such groups as the National Research Council of the National Academy of Sciences (<u>Risking the Future</u>, 1989), the Society for Adolescent Medicine, and the National Commission on the Role of the School and the Community in Improving Adolescent Health, which was jointly formed in 1989 by the American Medical Association and the National Association of State Boards of Education (<u>Code Blue: Uniting for Healthier Youth</u>).

A 1987 statement of the National PTA asserts that "(s)chool-linked health clinics are the only source of health care for many teens. They provide a wide variety of critical services such as immunizations, nutrition counseling, suicide prevention programs, drug and alcohol abuse prevention and treatment programs and general health assessments. By being on or near the school grounds, the health services are much more likely to be used." Most recently, in a report to Congress on Adolescent Health, the Office of Technology Assessment highlighted the importance of "school-linked or community-based centers that offer comprehensive and accessible services designed to meet adolescents' needs for physical accessibility, approachability, confidentiality and low or no cost."

The school-based clinic movement is truly a grass-roots movement. Communities recognizing that lack of adequate health care services threatens the future of their adolescents and seeking workable solutions have given significant momentum to the movement. The number of identified SBCs increased four-fold between 1984 and 1989, from 31 to 150. At the present time, CPO is aware of over 300 SBCs and school-linked clinics (SLCs) across the country.

School-linked and school-based clinics are not without their critics, however. Most of the criticism - and indeed, the strongest opposition - centers around the issue of family planning and contraceptive services and counselling. Since the results of CPO's evaluation of six school-based clinics (attached), there has been a steady stream of negative articles focusing on the lack of concrete evidence that SBCs reduce teen pregnancy. Much of what is written in these articles distorts the truth by leaving out information that does not support their views and by drawing conclusions which the data do not support.

Opponents of SBCs characterize them as "birth control programs" which promote value-free promiscuity among the students attending schools in which they are located. Nothing could be further from the truth. Some critics of SBCs confuse "correlation" with "causation". They cite examples of clinic schools with high pregnancy rates compared to schools without clinics with lower pregnancy rates and draw the conclusion that clinics promote promiscuity and therefore promoted increases in pregnancy rates. The more likely explanation is that SBCs are started in communities with high pregnancy rates as one way of addressing the problem. In CPO's study where comparison schools were matched on the basis of geographic, demographic and socio-economic characteristics, there were no differences between clinic and comparison schools in pregnancy rates.

Furthermore, the assumption that SBCs are primarily teen pregnancy prevention programs is a fundamental error. While the initial motivation for starting some clinics was the expectation that SBC programs would be able to address teen pregnancy as part of comprehensive medical care, family planning services are not the primary services being offered. Even in the few clinics where contraceptives are available on site, family planning visits comprise only about a quarter of the total visits.

The primary purpose of school-based clinics is to provide health care to a typically underserved population in an easily accessible location. To suggest that policymakers evaluate school-based clinics solely on the basis of school-wide pregnancy rates is ludicrous. CPO's evaluation of SBCs demonstrated that it is unrealistic to expect this intervention by itself to resolve the problem of adolescent pregnancy. SBCs, however, can serve as one important component of the multiple interventions needed to make a difference.

Only a small percentage of SBCs actually provide contraceptives on-site. The lack of access as well as the message of ambivalence this sends to sexually active students necessarily weakens the potential of the SBC's reproductive health services to prevent pregnancies. Where contraceptives are not available in the clinic, students are less likely to come to the clinic for reproductive health counseling. Opportunities for health providers to discuss responsible sexual decision-making -- including abstinence as a possible option -- with students are undoubtedly lost.

The provision of contraceptives on site does not result in an increase in the percentages of students who are sexually experienced, does not result in a decrease in the mean age at first intercourse among sexually experienced students, nor does it result in an increase in the frequency with which students engage in intercourse. In fact, in some sites where this has been assessed, there was evidence of less sexual activity among students attending the clinic schools compared to the non-clinic schools. The percentages of sexually experienced students in many schools is very high -- sometimes over 85% -- regardless of whether an SBC is

47-042 - 92 - 7

present or not. Sexually active students need access to adequate reproductive health care.

On the basis of its evaluation study, CPO was able to provide a set of recommendations which, if implemented, can improve the SBC's ability to address the issue of adolescent pregnancy more effectively. Some of these recommendations include: 1) giving a high priority to pregnancy and STD prevention ; 2) conducting more outreach into the school; 3) identifying and targeting students engaged in sexual activity; 4) making contraceptives available through the clinic; 5) implementing effective follow-up procedures; and 6) emphasizing condoms and male responsibility.

When the overwhelming majority - 84% - of teen pregnancies are unintended, it is clear that more effective prevention efforts are necessary. It is high time to reassess the strategies of the last decade. Teenagers need sexuality education that is both accurate and comprehensive in its discussion of birth control options, including abstinence. They need confidential access to family planning services and reproductive health care. And they need all this both before and after they become sexually active.

Reducing the rates of too-early childbearing in this country is within our reach. Education is one key to prevention; access to services is another. So too is a commitment to ensuring that all teenagers have access to comprehensive health care and real options for their futures. School-based and school-linked clinics are one of many strategies that show promise for achieving these goals.

By Douglas Kirby, Ph.D.
and Cynthia S. Waszak
with Julie Ziegler

An Assessment of Six School-Based Clinics: Services, Impact and Potential

Edited by Patricia Donovan

Center for Population Options
1012 14th Street, NW
Suite 1200
Washington, DC 20005
(202) 347-5700

Support Center for School-Based Clinics/CPO
5650 Kirby Drive
Suite 242
Houston, TX 77005
(713) 664-7400

Center for Population Options
The Center for Population Options (CPO) is a nonprofit educational organization dedicated to improving the quality of life for adolescents by preventing too-early childbearing.

CPO's national and international programs seek to improve adolescent decision-making through life planning and other educational programs, to improve access to reproductive health care, to promote the development of school-based clinics, and to prevent the spread among adolescents of HIV and other sexually transmitted diseases.

Table of Contents

Tables

Figures

Appendices

Acknowledgements

This evaluation relied heavily upon innumerable clinic practitioners, clinic administrators, school administrators, researchers, and teenagers. Their willingness to provide their support and share their time, knowledge, and data have greatly enhanced the comprehensiveness and validity of this study. The efforts of several groups should be emphasized.

Many people at each of the six sites contributed to this project. Most important, they agreed to have their programs scrutinized and evaluated by outside evaluators. They should be particularly commended for this openness. But they did much more than play a passive role. They also changed their clinic schedules so that we could meet with them; shared their insights into clinic operations with us; provided us with specially prepared summaries of clinic records; helped us obtain school approval to administer questionnaires to students; helped us actually administer those questionnaires; helped us understand the statistical results; and reviewed drafts of this report. Although numerous people at each site helped, some deserve special attention for their extra efforts:

Dallas:	Steven Rosser, Rick Scatterday, Truman Thomas
Gary:	Edna Brown, Jean Campbell, Mary Hicks
Jackson:	Ralph Burney, Maxine Orey, Aaron Shirley
Muskegon:	Mary Duskin, Jackie Stutesman, Nancy Windatt, Diann Fisher
Quincy:	Donna Barber, Sylvia Byrd, Meredieth M. Martin, Rita Rodgers, Phil Rond, Jerry Wynn
San Francisco:	Claire Brindis, Kim Cox, Laura Seltzer, Valerie Stoller, Geraldine Oliva

Claire Brindis deserves special mention, because she made all the arrangements for administering both the pretest and posttest health surveys in San Francisco, and then actually administered both those surveys.

This project is also heavily indebted to the thousands of teenagers who voluntarily participated in this research. The vast majority of them completed the health surveys thoughtfully and honestly. Some of them even completed the survey two or three times.

The research advisory board for this project contributed to the project's success. Although its membership evolved as the needs of the project evolved, all of the following people contributed important ideas based upon their different experience and perspectives:

Michael Baizerman
Marsha Beatty
Claire Brindis
Joy Dryfoos
Frank Furstenberg
Sandra Hofferth
Sharon Lovick
Lani Majer
Karen Pittman
Laurie Zabin

Also contributing to the review process were members of the advisory board for the Support Center for School-Based Clinics: Tom Berkshire, Guy Parcel, David Gurule, Victoria Thompkins, Georgia Macdonough, Diane Allensworth, Genie Wessel, Alwyn Cohall, and David Kaplan.

At the Center for Population Options, several people contributed greatly to this project. Julie Ziegler conducted all the statistical analysis. She helped administer the health survey, coordinated a massive amount of keypunching, and meticulously ran hundreds of computer programs. The statistical tables that she produced were voluminous.

Judith Senderowitz, Executive Director of the Center for Population Options, provided a great deal of support for this project, from the beginning to the end. She recognized the importance of evaluating school-based clinics, helped secure funding to conduct the evaluation, and provided both overall guidance and innumerable suggestions.

Sharon Lovick, Director of CPO's Support Center for School-Based Clinics, also provided support, overall direction and innumerable insights. Her vast experience working within clinics, directing a clinic, and providing technical assistance to other clinics were invaluable during the site visits and throughout the project. She helped us better understand the operation of clinics, the human factor behind some of the statistics, and the limitations of the quantitative data.

Finally, the Ford Foundation, the William T. Grant Foundation, and the Charles Stewart Mott Foundation provided the funding for diverse aspects of this project, including methods development and testing, data collection and analysis, and publication of the report. That funding was obviously critical to the completion of this work. The interpretations and conclusions contained in this publication represent the views of the authors and the Center for Population Options and not necessarily those of these Foundations, their Trustees, or officers.

Consequently, I wish to express my sincere appreciation to everyone who helped make this a successful project.

Douglas Kirby

CHAPTER 1

Executive Summary: Utilization, Impact, and Potential of School-Based Clinics

Since the first school-based health clinic opened in a Dallas high school in 1970, school-based clinics have been seen not only as a means of providing basic health care to medically underserved teenagers, but also as a promising way of addressing some of the increasingly intractable and complex health and social problems facing young people, particularly unintended pregnancy.*

Today, there are 150 school-based clinics (SBCs) operating in middle, junior, and senior high schools in most major cities as well as in many rural areas, usually with widespread public support.** These clinics, which often serve low-income, predominantly minority youth with limited access to other sources of health care, provide a wide range of medical and counseling services. Most provide primary health care, physical examinations, laboratory tests, diagnosis and treatment of illness and minor injuries, immunizations, gynecological exams, pregnancy testing and counseling, referral for prenatal care, birth control information and referral, nutrition education, weight reduction programs and counseling for substance abuse. Some offer prenatal care on site; a few dispense contraceptives and provide day care for children of students.

School-based clinics are well used by students in the schools they serve. On average, about half of the student body enrolls in the SBC—in some schools the proportion is much higher—and eight in 10 of those enrolled actually use the clinic's services. For about half of enrolled students, school-based clinics are their sole or primary source of health care (5).

As the SBC movement stands on the brink of its third decade, however, it is appropriate to assess more definitively than ever before the actual impact of these clinics on students' access to medical care and on their health-related behavior, and to gain a better understanding of the potential impact of school-based clinics and methods of enhancing their effectiveness and reaching that potential. Perhaps excitement over the promise of school-based clinics led to unrealistic expectations of what these clinics, by themselves, could accomplish, particularly in influencing students' risk-taking behavior.

With these objectives in mind, the Center for Population Options (CPO) in 1984 launched a major project designed to evaluate a diverse group of clinics located in different parts of the country. The project sought to assess the students' utilization of clinic services and the clinics' impact on use of medical services generally. It also sought to determine what, if any, effect the clinics had on students' absenteeism, illegal drug use,

---

* The National Research Council of the National Academy of Sciences, for example, has called comprehensive health clinics in schools with large, high-risk populations a most promising approach to pregnancy prevention (1). Similarly, the Office of Technology Assessment has recommended the development of comprehensive school-based clinics in order to reduce high-risk pregnancies among teenagers (2). Such prominent organizations as the National Parent Teacher Association, the American Academy of Pediatrics, the National Education Association, the American College of Obstetricians and Gynecologists and the Association of School Nurses have publicly supported school-based clinics.

** Polls in Michigan and Oregon, for example, show that 77-80 percent of adults favor school-based clinics and that support is highest among parents of public school children (3). And nearly four out of five adults surveyed in North and South Carolina favor the establishment of school-based clinics (4).

alcohol consumption, cigarette smoking, and unprotected sexual intercourse, focusing particular attention on students' contraceptive use and the clinics' success in preventing unintended pregnancies. Finally, the study sought to examine clinics' potential to better meet their desired objectives and to identify ways they could do so. The findings of this five-year research project, are presented in this report. Included in this executive summary is a brief review of the principal factors that contributed to the development of school-based clinics and the current status of the school-based clinic movement, and following the summary of the findings, a discussion of their implications, and recommendations for making clinics more effective.

School-Based Clinics: A New Approach

Public schools have been involved in efforts to improve student health since before the turn of the century. Until recently, however, school health services were largely limited to health inspection, screening and assessment, and first aid provided by nurses, who, because of nursing practice regulations were unable to provide direct medical care or to prescribe and dispense medications.

Student health services in some schools began to change in the 1960s as a result both of the growing recognition that adolescents, in particular, needed better access to health care and of an increased commitment on the part of government and private foundations to the provision of health and social services to disadvantaged populations. Efforts to develop innovative health programs accelerated in the succeeding 10-20 years in response to several major developments:

- A dramatic increase in the number of single-parent households. In 1985, 22% of families with children under 18 were headed by a single parent (6). Twenty-four percent of children under age 18 lived in single-parent households; another 3% (1.9 million children) lived with neither parent (7).
- A large increase in the number of children living in poor families. More than 20% of all children under the age of 18 now live in families whose income is below the federal poverty level ($12,100 for a family of four) (8), and some 44% of these children live in families with incomes below half of the poverty standard (9).
- Rapid increases in health care costs at a time when the number of families with no medical insurance also increased. In 1984, 14% (4.5 million) of all 10-18 year olds had no health insurance (10).
- An increase in public awareness of and concern about the country's high rates of teenage pregnancy. About one million teenage girls become pregnant in the United States each year; some 416,000 of these teens terminate their pregnancies by abortion and roughly 480,000 give birth.* (The remaining pregnancies are miscarried or result in stillbirths (11).) These rates are significantly higher than rates in other western industrialized countries, despite similar levels of adolescent sexual activity (12).
- Widespread use of illegal drugs among adolescents. Although drug use appeared to have declined slightly, at least among high school seniors (13), it remains a serious problem, as does consumption of alcohol among teenagers.** Furthermore, the emerging crack problem may have serious, but as yet not fully understood, consequences for adolescents.

In the face of these developments, comprehensive health clinics—located on school campuses, staffed by health professionals trained in working with teenagers, and able to provide services at nominal or no charge—came to be viewed as a promising approach to addressing the increasingly complex health-care needs of adolescents. Now, the threat posed by AIDS (acquired immunodeficiency syndrome), along with rising rates of other

* These births typically have a negative impact on the teen mothers' lives in terms of education, job opportunities and the ability to stay off of welfare, and they also have a serious impact on society: Three federal poverty programs—Aid to Families with Dependent Children (AFDC), food stamps and Medicaid—together spend more than $19 billion annually to help families in which the mother gave birth as a teenager (14).

** About 40% of all teenage deaths are the result of automobile accidents (15), many of which involve teenage drivers who have been drinking. About one-quarter of eighth graders and more than a third of tenth graders report having had five or more drinks on at least one occasion (16).

sexually transmitted diseases (STDs) among teenagers, has added new urgency to the effort to provide adolescents with information to help them avoid risk-taking behavior, together with medical services to identify and address health problems that arise as a result of such behavior.

The appeal of school-based clinics has been bolstered by the realization that many teens do not receive adequate medical attention and are forced to rely heavily on more costly services of hospital emergency rooms when problems arise. These emergency rooms can treat serious illnesses and injuries, but do not provide on-going preventive medical care or health education and do not treat emotional and psychological problems unless they are severe. Some 15% of 16- and 17-year-olds have no regular source of medical care (17).

To a great extent, this inadequate health care is probably a consequence of the high cost of medical care and the widespread lack of insurance. However, it also reflects the fact that scheduling doctor visits has become a problem in this era of single-parent and two-working-parent households. Doctors' offices and health clinics normally are not open in the evenings and on weekends, and working parents often have difficulty arranging to leave their jobs to take their children to a doctor during the day. Furthermore, while increasing numbers of pediatricians have had some training in adolescent medicine, teenagers are often treated by physicians, whether pediatricians or adults' doctors, who are ill-equipped to deal with many of the sensitive issues that concern adolescents, particularly those relating to sexual development.

School-based clinics that provide comprehensive primary health care can address many of these problems of access because they do not require parents to arrange to take their child to a doctor; they offer confidential* services free or at low cost, often without a prearranged appointment; and they employ nurse practitioners, doctors and counselors who are skilled at identifying and treating physical as well as emotional and psychological problems that students often face.

School-Based Clinics in 1989

According to CPO's latest survey of school-based clinics, conducted in the spring of 1989 by its Support Center for School-Based Clinics, there are currently 150 school-based clinics operated by a total of 90 programs, most of which are traditional providers of medical care—hospitals and medical schools, public health departments, nonprofit organizations, and community health clinics; however, an increasing number of clinics (currently 20%) are operated directly by school districts (see Table 1.1). The number of clinics has increased five-fold since 1983 (18).

Table 1.1
Percentages of school-based clinics (N=130) by type of sponsoring agency, according to recent survey results

Type of agency	Percentage
Hospital/medical school	26
Nonprofit organization	19
Community clinic	12
Public health clinic	23
School system	20

Clinics are now located in 32 states and in 91 communities. Most operate in senior high schools, although 14% are in junior high or middle schools. Schools with school-based clinics have an average enrollment of about 1300 students, although the size of the student body ranges from 224 to 3627. On the average, 48% of students in clinic schools are enrolled in the clinic and thereby eligible to receive services, and 80% of those enrolled use the clinic at some point during the year.

A majority of clinics are open at least 40 hours a week, although the proportion declined from 76% in 1988 to 66% in 1989. Almost 90% of clinics operate every weekday, and more than half remain open during the summer, although these percentages also dropped somewhat from 1988 to 1989. These declines reflect decreases in funding, which force clinics to use fewer staff and to shorten their hours of operation [see Box: top of next page].

* Virtually all clinics require students to have parental consent to enroll in the program; some seek blanket permission to provide all services, others give parents the opportunity to indicate which services their children may, or may not, receive. State law, however, often permits certain services, such as family planning, treatment for sexually transmitted diseases (STDs) and drug and alcohol abuse counseling, to be provided without parental consent, and some clinics do not require parental consent for these services.

FUNDING FOR SCHOOL-BASED CLINICS

School-based clinics are funded by a variety of public and private sources. In 1989, about two-thirds of SBC funding came from public sources: the states accounted for 19% of total funding; cities and counties contributed 16%; and the Maternal and Child Health Block Grant also provided about 16% of clinic funding. Medicaid, the Early and Periodic Screening, Diagnosis and Treatment (EPSDT) program and the Community Health Services Block Grant each provided between 2 and 4% of total funding. School districts contributed about three percent.

Foundations are virtually the only source of private funding for school-based clinics. In 1989, foundations provided 31% of total funding, down from 41% the previous year. Insurance payments and patient fees each accounted for less than one percent of clinic funding.

Most clinics were funded by at least two sources, and about half by at least three. Clinics also received in-kind contributions, primarily in the form of facilities, utilities and maintenance. The value of in-kind support ranged from $4,700 to $137,000 and averaged about $35,000.

SBC operating budgets averaged $125,000 in 1989, although they ranged from $100,000 to $313,000. As would be expected, the average varied substantially depending on the clinic's hours of operation. Clinics open less than 20 hours a week had an average operating budget of $43,000, while a clinic open 40 hours had an average budget of $142,000. Clinics that had been open less than a year had higher budgets than those that had been operating for three years, reflecting higher one-time start-up costs.

Clinic Users

Fifty-nine percent of all clinic users are black (up from 49% in 1988). This reflects the fact that school-based clinics typically serve low-income areas, which tend to be disproportionately populated by minorities. About one-quarter of users are white, and 12% are Hispanic. On the average, 38% of clinic users are male. Males are typically a difficult group to reach with adolescent health services. One recent study, however, found that school-based clinics saw a larger proportion of males than did other adolescent health programs (19). About one-third of school-based clinic users have no health insurance.

Most clinics limit eligibility for services to students enrolled in the school in which they are located, but some also are open to dropouts (16%), children of students (16%), other family members of students (11%), and adolescents in the broader community (9%).

Clinic Services

The average clinic serves 59 students and handles about 183 visits each month. Table 1.2 shows the broad array of services that school-based clinics provide. For the most part, this list has changed little in the past few years, but there have been some notable changes in the proportion of clinics offering certain services, particularly in the area of reproductive health care: only 15% currently dispense contraceptives, compared with 28% in 1986, and the proportion that prescribe contraceptives declined from 52% to 40% over the same time period. Whereas, 20% of clinics referred students to family planning agencies for birth control in 1986 (20), almost three quarters do so now. It thus appears that despite widespread public support for providing contraceptives in school-based clinics,* few of the clinics that have opened in recent years have decided to dispense contraceptives.

The proportion of clinics offering prenatal care also has dropped markedly, from 47% in 1987 (21) to 30% in 1989; however, 94% of clinics refer pregnant students for prenatal services. There have been smaller declines in the past year in the percentages of clinics providing drug and substance abuse counseling, weight reduction programs, gynecological exams and mental health and psychosocial counseling. These declines are not considered significant, however, because newer programs tend to add these programs after the first year or so of operation, and the decline reflects the addition of many new programs.

Past Research on Clinic Effectiveness

This statistical information provides valuable data on how school-based clinics are currently operating and whom they are serving, but it does not assess clinics' effectiveness in delivering services and in enabling students to avoid unplanned pregnancies and risk-taking behaviors.

Perhaps because most of the growth in school-based clinics has occurred in the last few years, there has been little research on the clinics' impact on student health and

* A 1988 Harris Poll, for example, indicates that 80% of adults favor making birth control information and contraceptives available in school-based clinics (22).

Table 1.2
Percentages of school-based clinics (N=92) currently providing various services, according to recent survey results

Services provided	Percentages
Medical services	
Sports/work physicals	98
Diagnosis and treatment of minor injuries	97
General primary health care	96
Lab tests	96
Prescribe medication	96
Assessment or referrals to local physicians	93
Assessment or referrals to community health care	92
General physicals	91
Immunizations	89
Chronic illness management	75
Dispense medication	74
EPSDT screening	54
Dental services	34
Pediatric care for infants	29
Counseling/educational services	
Health education	98
Nutrition education	96
Mental health/psychosocial counseling	89
Pregnancy counseling	83
Sexuality education in class	83
Weight reduction programs	79
Family counseling with student and parents	62
Drug/substance abuse programs	61
Job counseling	25
Reproductive health and family planning services	
Referrals for prenatal care	93
Pregnancy tests	88
Counseling on birth control methods	85
Diagnosis/treatment of STDs	78
Gynecological exams	77
Referrals for birth control methods and exams	72
Follow-up for birth control users	71
Exams for selected birth control methods	55
Prescriptions for birth control methods	43
Prenatal care on-site	28
Dispensation of birth control methods	12
Other activities	
AIDS education program in class	38
AIDS education program in clinic	34
Day care for children of students	15

behavior. However, studies that have been done provide some evidence that clinics can have a positive impact in this area. For example, a student survey conducted two years after the opening of a school-based clinic in a Kansas City, Missouri high school found that 55% of clinic users who were sexually active used some form of birth control, compared with only 35% of sexually active students who did not use the clinic (23). An analysis of the effect of school-based clinic use on adolescent contraceptive behavior among students at a large urban high school in Texas found that clinic users were twice as likely to use contraception every time they had sex, compared with students who had not been to the clinic. Furthermore, clinic users were less than half as likely to have never used a birth control method. Of course, there may have been self-selection effects — students who were sufficiently motivated to use the clinic for contraception also might have obtained it elsewhere if the clinic had not been present. The researchers concluded, however, that "a number of factors may influence an adolescent's decision to seek preventive health or reproductive services, but, at the least, school-based clinics may enable students to carry out preventive intentions and to avoid an unplanned pregnancy (24)."

Stronger evidence was found in a study comparing an experimental pregnancy prevention program that combined classroom presentations and counseling in two inner-city Baltimore schools with reproductive health services provided to the students at a nearby clinic. Significantly lower pregnancy rates were found among the experimental program participants. Over a period of nearly three years, the pregnancy rate declined 30% among students in the program schools — one junior high and one senior high — while it increased 58% in two control schools. In addition, there was an average delay of almost seven months in the initiation of sexual intercourse among the program-school students, and younger students in the experimental schools were much more likely than those in the control schools to use contraception. Although technically not a school-based clinic (medical services were not provided in the school itself and the clinic provided only reproductive health care), the program's evaluators concluded that access to high quality, free services, professional counseling, education, and open communication — all key elements of a good school-based clinic — were important to the program's success: "All these factors appear to have created an atmosphere that allowed teenagers to translate their attitudes into constructive preventive behavior (25)."

Reported declines in fertility rates among students in high schools participating in the school-based clinic program in St. Paul, Minnesota, (26), are often cited as evidence of the positive impact of SBCs. It is not clear, however, how great an impact the program had on the early large decline in birthrates because there was only one year of baseline data for the period before the program began, the data were dependent upon program personnel's knowledge of births among students, and because abortion data were not available.

Other studies have provided data on other health problems. For example, one study reported that a clinic in West Dallas detected previously undiagnosed health problems, including such potentially serious conditions as heart murmurs, in 30% of the students who attended the clinic (27). Another study reported that 32% of Pap smears taken at two school-based clinics in New York City were found to be abnormal during a four-month period (28).

Six School-Based Clinics: An In-Depth Evaluation

Given the rapid recent proliferation of school-based clinics, and given the fact that SBCs are often cited as an effective way of addressing some of adolescents' most serious health and social problems, the Center for Population Options believed more information was needed on the actual effect of school-based clinics on students' use of medical care, absenteeism, and their impact on risk-taking behaviors, such as smoking, drinking, illegal drug use, and unprotected sexual intercourse (including contraceptive use and pregnancy). CPO also thought it was important to understand the barriers to effective delivery of services and the potential for improving clinics' effectiveness. Recognizing that a study of multiple sites would allow greater generalization of the findings to other school-based clinics than would an analysis of a single clinic, CPO selected six clinics for in-depth evaluation. These clinics were chosen because they met predetermined criteria regarding size of population served, logistical considerations, nonparticipation in other evaluation projects and the sites' interest in participating. Although these clinics account for only 4% of the total number of clinics currently operating, and although the clinics may have increased their effectiveness since the last data were collected in 1987 and 1988, the study nonetheless sheds light on the areas where school-based clinics have had or can have a positive impact, as well as on the areas where clinics are not likely to have as much of an effect as had originally been expected.

The clinics selected for evaluation were in Gary, Indiana; Muskegon, Michigan; Jackson, Mississippi; Dallas, Texas; Quincy, Florida; and San Francisco, California. All six clinics served low-income populations, provided primary health care, and were open daily during school hours. In a number of important respects, however, they differed from each other. The Dallas clinic, for example, is the country's oldest SBC, having opened its doors in 1970. The San Francisco and Quincy clinics, on the other hand, had not opened when the research project began. The clinics also varied significantly in size, ranging from 1,600 visits annually in the Gary clinic to 10,500 visits (including students from schools other than the clinic site) in Dallas, which was the only one of the clinics studied that serves teenagers who did not attend the home school.* In five of the six schools, the students were predominantly black, but the San Francisco student body was a mixture of black, Hispanic and Asian students. The clinics also varied in their principal goals and objectives; some, for example, stressed pregnancy prevention, while others did not.

To evaluate each clinic, it was necessary to have some means of comparing student populations in schools with clinics to student populations without access to clinic programs. For each of the four clinics operating at the initiation of the project — Gary, Muskegon, Jackson, and Dallas — comparison schools were identified that were as similar as possible to the clinic schools in terms of relevant sociodemographic characteristics and as physically close as possible. Since clinics had not yet opened in the Quincy and San Francisco schools when the study began, baseline data on variables of interest could be collected and compared with data gathered after the clinic had been operating for two years. Data used in the evaluation were drawn from four sources, which together present a coherent and consistent picture of school-based clinics. The sources were:

■ **Interviews with school and clinic staff and students** conducted throughout the course of the project, which provided general information about the school and its clinic.

■ **Records from each of the clinics**, which, though they varied from computerized encounter forms to handwritten logs, were all able to provide data on the number of clinic

* The clinic is part of the Children and Youth Project administered by the University of Texas Health Science Center. It serves adolescents aged 12-18 in the community regardless of whether they attend the clinic school.

users and their sociodemographic characteristics; the number of clinic visits per user and diagnoses made at each visit; the number of lab tests and referrals made; the number and type of family planning visits; and, depending on the particular clinic, the number of students referred either for contraception or the number given prescriptions or contraceptives.

■ **A Student Health Survey**, administered to a sample of students at both the clinic and comparison schools, which provided data on the impact of school-based clinics on students' attitudes and behaviors related to seeking medical services, risk-taking, and pregnancy prevention.

■ **Longitudinal birthrate data**, which were collected in two sites — Gary and Muskegon — to assess those clinics' impact on birthrates. In Gary, comparisons could be made between the clinic and non-clinic schools over an eight-year period. In Muskegon, birthrates at the clinic school over a seven-year period before and after the school clinic opened were compared.

Survey and birthrate methods was used in this study assessed the clinics' impact upon the entire student body, and not specifically upon those who actually used the clinic. Comparisons between clinic users and nonusers in terms of clinic impact have the disadvantage of possible selection bias due to the different characteristics and motivations of students who choose to use the clinic and those who do not. Because it is impossible to randomly assign students to school-based clinic services, this is a difficulty that cannot be resolved in this type of evaluation. In addition, although the sample sizes were quite large, they were not sufficiently large to detect small changes or changes in infrequently occurring outcomes, such as pregnancy. Finally, all self-report data are always open to the criticism that they are not reliable or valid, but there is evidence presented in this report that the data were reliable in most cases.

Findings

Clinic Utilization

One measure of the effectiveness of school-based clinics is the extent to which they are used by the students. Clinic use was measured in terms of the percentage of students visiting the clinic in a single year; the percentage of the students who ever had visited the clinic; and the number of visits per student.

Clinic use. Clinic use was highest in Dallas and Muskegon, where 80% and 70% of the student body, respectively, attended the clinic in a single year, and 83% and 82% ever had visited the clinic. About two thirds of the students in Quincy and Jackson used the clinics in a single year, while one quarter did so in San Francisco and Gary; again, the percentages who had ever used the clinic were higher than the single-year percentages in each of these schools. Moreover, the longer the students had been in the school, the more likely they were to have used the clinic. In Dallas, for example, 74% of first-year students and 89% of fourth-year students had used the clinic at some point. And the proportion of students ever using the San Francisco clinic increased from 40% at the end of the first year to 50% at the end of the second. This is undoubtedly because the longer students had attended the clinic school, the more opportunities they had to learn about the clinic, both from the staff in classroom presentations and through other "official" channels, and also from friends and classmates. They also had a longer period of time in which a need for medical care could have arisen.

Number of clinic visits. Many students who used the clinic did so only once or twice during the course of a year: in four sites that could provide information on visits per student in a single year, more than half of the users visited the clinic no more than three times a year. Similarly, the health survey indicated that most students who had ever used the clinic had done so infrequently; however, between 8% and 29% of users had visited the clinic a total of at least eight times, and could be considered "core" users.

Clinic users. The clinics served a greater percentage of females (53% to 64% of students at each sight) than males; clinic users were overwhelmingly black, except in San Francisco, where clinic users were more equally divided among blacks, Hispanics, and Asians; and users were concentrated among 16- and 17-year-olds. In each case, the proportions generally reflected the composition of the student body. A majority of clinic users came from low-income and/or single- or no-parent households; between 48% and 68% lived with one or neither parent, for example, and 6% to 40% of users' families received food stamps.

Clinic services. There were various services offered to students at different sites. All clinics offered some primary care (first aid/emergency care and treatment of sickness), but they varied in the extent to which they addressed reproductive health. All provided contraceptive counseling, for example, but this service was used most widely at the four clinics — Muskegon, Jackson, Dallas, and Quincy — that also dispensed or provided vouchers for contraceptives. Seventeen to 26 percent of all students surveyed at these four schools used the clinic to obtain contraceptives, and according to clinic records at those sites, family planning visits comprised 24% to 28% of their total visits. At the two clinics that did not provide contraceptives, very few students (3% to 5%) used the clinics for contraceptive counseling and referrals.

Some clinics provided preventive care in the form of general health assessments or health maintenance exams, screened for specific problems, such as high blood pressure, and offered assistance with nutrition and weight control. All made referrals for dental care, and the Dallas clinic provided regular dental services on site.

Reasons for clinic use and non-use. Users cited easy access and their relationship with the staff as their chief reasons for using the clinic. Specifically, the three most often cited reasons were: the clinic was part of the school and they felt they could trust it; the clinic was easy to get to; and the staff was caring. Students who cited one of these reasons used the clinic more frequently and for a greater variety of services than students who did not cite these reasons for use.

Lack of need was the principal explanation students gave for never having visited the clinic; it was cited by 43% to 87% of nonusers. In addition, some students didn't feel comfortable at the clinic, and others were concerned about confidentiality. Six to 27 percent said they "just didn't get around" to going to the clinic.

Impact on Utilization of Medical Care

To determine whether the presence of a school-based clinic affects students' overall utilization of medical care, comparisons were made between each of the six clinic-school samples and their non-clinic-school counterparts on the length of time that had elapsed since students had seen a doctor or a dentist, and whether they had visited an emergency room or had been hospitalized during the past year. Information gathered in Dallas and Quincy concerning how recently students had had a physical examination or routine lab tests were analyzed as well.

Doctor visits. The same percentages of clinic- and comparison-school students at each site (roughly two-thirds to three-quarters) had seen a physician within the previous 12 months, and between 79% and 93% had done so within the last two years. Only the Dallas clinic, which was the only clinic in the study that employed a full-time physician and which arranged for all students to receive an examination when they first entered the school, had an impact on how likely the students were to have seen a doctor recently; 72% of students in the clinic school, but only 61% of the students in the comparison school, had seen a doctor within the previous 12 months.

Lab tests/examinations. Also in Dallas, a larger percentage of students in the clinic school than in the comparison school had received a physical examination, a blood test, and a urine test within the last two years, although the proportions were high in both schools, ranging from 70% to 86%. And in Quincy, the only other site where these services were measured, there also was a significant increase in the percentage of students who had recently had a urine test after the clinic had been operating for two years, but there was not a significant increase in the percentages of students who had received a blood test or physical examination.

Dental care. In two sites — Muskegon and Dallas — the students in the clinic schools had seen a dentist more recently than in the comparison schools. The Dallas clinic provided dental care on site, while the Muskegon clinic made referrals for dental care. In the remaining four sites, however, no differences wee found.

Given the significant impact of the school-based clinic on health care received by students in Dallas, in terms of visits to a doctor and a dentist, physical examinations and laboratory tests, it seems likely that clinics that have a large staff, offer a wide array of services, and made a concerted effort to bring students into the clinic would have greater impact on students' receipt of health care than clinics that do not meet these conditions.

Hospital care. Experts have differed in their expectations for the impact of school-based clinics on visits to emergency rooms and nights spent in the hospital. Some have argued that clinics could reduce the need for these types of care, but others have contended that students use these services primarily for serious health problems, such as injuries and acute illness, that could not be prevented or treated by the school-based clinics. The results of this evaluation provide support for the latter view. There were no significant differences between the clinic and non-clinic samples in terms of either emergency room visits or hospitalization.

Impact on Risk-taking and Pregnancy Prevention

The evaluation sought to determine the potential of school-based clinics to reduce students' absenteeism, use of cigarettes, alcohol, and illegal drugs and to encourage the use of contraception among sexually active teens.

Absenteeism. In Quincy and San Francisco, according to survey results, significantly fewer days were missed due to illness two years after the opening of the clinic, though this difference amounted to about half a day over a four-week period. No significant differences were found between the clinic and non-clinic schools in Gary, Muskegon and Jackson, while in Dallas, students in the clinic school missed more days than their non-clinic counterparts. An analysis of school attendance records in Quincy indicated that while there were fewer absences due to illness after the clinic opened, the overall rate of absenteeism (including absences for reasons other than illness) did not decrease. There was no significant decrease in the number of days skipped (non-excused absences) for any of the clinic schools surveyed compared to their non-clinic or pre-clinic counterparts.

Cigarette smoking, alcohol consumption and drug use. At three of the four sites where alcohol consumption was measured, the frequency of consumption was significantly lower at the clinic school than in its non-clinic counterpart; most of these differences were in the percentages of students who never or rarely drank. No significant difference in alcohol consumption was found in the fourth site. In one of these sites, where students at the clinic school underwent a psychosocial assessment at their first clinic visit designed to identify students who engaged in risk-taking behaviors and might therefore need counseling, students also smoked less frequently than students in the comparison school. There were no differences between the clinic and non-clinic samples in the frequency of use of illegal drugs at the two sites where this activity was measured. However, it is difficult to assess the true extent of illegal drug use through self-report, since many students may not answer this question truthfully.

Sexual activity. Opponents of school-based clinics frequently charge that clinics that dispense or prescribe contraceptives promote sexual activity among students. This criticism is not supported by the results of this evaluation; the clinics did not hasten the initiation of sexual intercourse, nor increase its frequency among sexually active students. None of the clinic schools had a significantly higher percentage of sexually active students than did their comparison schools, and sexually active students in the clinic schools did not have sex more frequently than their counterparts in the comparison schools. To the contrary, one of the clinic schools, Muskegon, had a smaller percentage of students who had ever had sex; sexually active students in two of the clinic schools, Jackson and Dallas, had sex for the first time at an older age than did the students in the comparison schools; and sexually active students in the San Francisco school reported less frequent sexual intercourse two years after the clinic opened than before the clinic opened.

Contraceptive use. At two of the six sites—Muskegon and San Francisco—significantly more students in the clinic-school samples than in the non-clinic-school or pre-clinic-school samples used some type of contraception at last intercourse. At both sites, this difference was due primarily to increased condom use, and to a lesser extent, birth control pill use, since clinic-school students at these sites were also more likely than their non-clinic-school counterparts to have used either birth control pills or condoms (rather than less effective methods such as withdrawal, rhythm or foam) the last time they had intercourse.

The Muskegon clinic transferred student records to a nearby Planned Parenthood clinic and provided vouchers for contraceptives to be redeemed free of charge there. The San Francisco clinic neither prescribed nor dispensed contraceptives, but provided contraceptive counseling and referrals. Notably, both clinics had aggressive outreach into the school to provide contraceptive education. In San Francisco, where there was a salient threat of AIDS, there were several programs developed through the clinic to make students aware of the need to use condoms. Students from this school also were exposed to intensive city wide media campaigns promoting condom use.

In Gary, Jackson, Dallas and Quincy, no differences were found in the use of condoms or pills at last intercourse between the clinic and non-clinic samples. At the sites dispensing contraceptives or making vouchers available — Jackson, Muskegon, Dallas and Quincy — students who had ever used the clinic for contraception were more likely to use either condoms or pills at last intercourse than were those students who had never used the clinic for this purpose. The same self-selection effects identified in earlier studies applies for this last analysis as well, however.

Sexually active students in both clinic and non-clinic schools, who were asked for all reasons why they had not always used contraception during intercourse, most often said they didn't expect to have sex (21% to 57% cited this reason) and they didn't think pregnancy would occur (cited by 14% to 42% percent). Discomfort in going to a strange clinic, a partner's desire not to use contraception and apathy were other common explanations for their behavior. Students who cited these reasons for not practicing contraception were in fact, more likely not to practice contraception at last intercourse than students who did not check these reasons.

Pregnancy and birthrates. There were no differences among students at the clinic and non-clinic schools at any of the six sites as to whether they had been pregnant or gotten someone pregnant within the last 12 months. These results should be viewed cautiously, however, because some teenagers who conceived while in high school subsequently may have dropped out and not been present to complete the Student Health Survey, and other teenagers may not have reported previous pregnancies. However, this underreporting should not have differentially affected the results from the clinic-school and non- or pre-clinic-school samples surveyed.

Birthrates were calculated in two sites—Gary and Muskegon. In the former, there were variations in birthrates over time, but the rates varied similarly for both the clinic and control schools, indicating that the school-based clinic had no impact on birthrates. In Muskegon, comparisons were made in the birthrates at the clinic school before and after the clinic opened. Although there was a decline in the birthrate over time, it is not possible to determine from the available data whether the decline was more rapid after the clinic opened than before it opened.

Summary and Recommendations

The primary purpose of school-based clinics is to provide young people, many of whom have no other regular source of medical care, with comprehensive health care, and this evaluation indicates that these clinics were successful in achieving this objective. Very large percentages of students used the clinic in five of the schools studied, and in the sixth clinic, the proportion of users increased each year after it opened. Most students used the school-based clinic infrequently, primarily for treatment for illness, first aid, physical exams and counseling; however, a small core group of students used the clinic considerably more often, and it was these students upon whom clinics may have had their most significant impact. Easy access to the clinic and trust in its staff were the key factors that encouraged students to use a school-based clinic. Most non-use appears to be related to lack of need, but some students did not use a school-based clinic because they were concerned about confidentiality or because they "just didn't get around to it." These clinics must devise ways to allay such concerns and to motivate students in need to take advantage of their services.

Since most communities have alternative sources of health care available, a key question is whether school-based clinics actually increase students' access to health care or simply replace providers that were used in the past. While substitution did occur, the study findings indicate that the more resources these clinics had, the greater their impact on access: more students saw doctors and dentists in the clinic where those professionals were employed full-time, and more students received health maintenance exams when those exams were a routine part of the clinic program. However, the question of impact on access cannot be fully answered on the basis of the results from this study, in part because of the questions asked. In most clinics, including most of those evaluated in this project, the primary health care provider is a nurse or nurse practitioner, not a doctor, so that fewer doctor visits cannot be equated with less care.

Future studies should build on what was learned in this evaluation by asking more specific questions about the types of health care workers seen and the frequency with which specific health needs such as minor illness, injury and treatment for STDs are unmet. To determine the impact of school-based clinics on emergency room and hospital admissions, it may also be helpful to examine the impact on emergency room use for different health reasons. Many admissions may be due to causes that could not possibly be prevented by clinics, while other causes may be preventable. It may also be helpful to examine students' perceptions of the role of school-based clinics in the context of other sources of medical care available to them in their communities.

The study provides encouraging indications that school-based clinics can reduce students' consumption of alcohol and tobacco. The impact on both smoking and drinking depends partially on educational efforts, and the evaluation results demonstrate the potential for school-based clinic intervention in this area.

The results of this study demonstrate that these school-based clinics did not encourage students to be sexually active, even when the clinic dispensed or prescribed contraceptives. Moreover, users of clinics that dispensed contraceptives were more likely than non-users in the same school to use birth control and to use effective methods of contraception.

The results also indicate, however, that providing contraceptives is not enough, by itself, to significantly increase contraceptive use among sexually active students in the entire school. The findings that the school-based clinic samples in Dallas, Jackson, and Quincy (which provided contraceptives) did not have higher rates of contraceptive use than their non-clinic school counterparts, and that the San Francisco clinic sample had higher rates of condom use than the pre-clinic sample even though it did not prescribe or dispense contraceptives, suggests that school-based clinics should provide contraceptive information as well as physical access to contraceptives. Community-wide intensive education campaigns, such as those mounted in San Francisco during the AIDS crisis, may motivate students to find sources of contraception, even if these sources are outside of the school. The physical availability of contraceptives within the school does not automatically provide greater incentive to use them, as is clear in those sites where the clinic dispensed birth control products but did little in the way of educational outreach or follow-up of patients and did not significantly increase contraceptive use.

According to survey data, school-based clinics had no effect on pregnancy rates. The birth rate did decline in one of the two schools where rates were measured, but the data varied from year to year and did not provide a conclusive explanation for why this occurred. The potential impact of school-based clinics on pregnancy and birthrates must continue to be studied, and in particular, should be assessed in connection with program changes described below that are designed to address these outcomes.

Improving Clinic Effectiveness

Clinics can take a number of steps to enhance their effectiveness in preventing pregnancies among students and in reducing risk-taking in other areas. Some of the recommendations that follow have already been implemented in some clinics. In many cases where they have not, implementation will require additional resources, which are often difficult to generate. Even with adequate resources and effective strategies, however, clinics face a difficult task in trying to alter students' risk-taking behaviors, many of which are deeply rooted in the values and practices of the larger community in which they live. Recommendations include:

- **Identify and target students engaged in risk-taking behaviors.** Clinics generally do a good job of treating and counseling students who seek their services, but they rarely have aggressive programs to identify risk-taking teens who are not motivated to come to the clinic. Scheduling routine physical examinations for all incoming students or administering psychosocial assessments can help clinics identify risk-takers. Clinics could also urge teachers and other personnel to refer risk-taking youth to them.
- **Provide comprehensive reproductive health services.** This evaluation demonstrated that students were far more likely to use a school-based clinic for reproductive health care if the clinic prescribed or dispensed contraceptives as well as offered counseling about birth control methods and pregnancy testing. Intensive education efforts, both in the clinic and in the classroom, are also critical. (Some possible approaches are discussed below).
- **Appointments for family planning counseling and for birth control should be offered promptly,** ideally on a walk-in basis, because teens are impulsive and may not be willing to wait a week or longer to make important decisions about sex (or other risk-taking behaviors). Clinics also need to follow up family planning patients more effectively in order to improve contraceptive continuation rates.
- **Reproductive health programs should place greater emphasis on male responsibility.** The findings in San Francisco and Muskegon suggest that it is possible to increase the use of condoms by males. Males have been much less likely than females to visit a school-based clinic for contraceptives, but they can be reached through sports physicals, classroom activities, and the media.
- **Conduct more outreach in the school.** Since most students use school-based clinics infrequently, it is important for clinics to undertake outreach efforts to provide teens with information and support that will help them avoid or discontinue risk-taking behavior. In the area of sexuality, clinics can work with the school to implement and participate in a comprehensive sexuality education program. In addition, clinics can place posters about the clinic and health-related topics throughout the school; write a regular column in the school newspaper; and make presentations at school assemblies.
- **Group sessions facilitated by trained clinic staff can provide students with more opportunities** to resolve difficult personal dilemmas about sex and other risk-taking behaviors, and at the same time, help students become familiar with clinic staff.
- **Develop community-wide programs.** School-based clinics cannot effectively address any difficult social problem in isolation. They need to involve the broader community, including parents, youth-serving agencies, religious and other community leaders, and the media.
- **Increase permanent staff.** Many clinics will need additional staff to implement the strategies proposed here. They also need to maintain staff continuity. To save money, some clinics use rotating physicians from nearby medical schools. Others pay low wages and lose full-time staff once they have gained sufficient experience to command higher

salaries elsewhere. Still others reassign more experienced staff to several schools or community health clinics in order to take wider advantage of their skills. Staff turnover reduces the continuity of the relationships that can be developed between the clinic and students.

■ **Provide education and deliver services earlier.** The results of this study indicate that many students were sexually active before entering high school. Where it is possible, programs operating school-based clinics should begin interventions in junior high or middle schools. These interventions should include effective peer-led programs to promote delayed sexual activity.

■ **Provide greater motivation for delaying pregnancy.** Some sexually active students were not highly motivated to avoid pregnancy. One possible way of providing this motivation may be by presenting pregnancy prevention messages within the context of a life planning curriculum, where students are encouraged to extend their education and begin a career before beginning a family. Also important is the provision of role models and improved job opportunities for youth in their communities.

School-based clinics have been successful in their short lifespan in providing primary and preventive care to the students they serve. Their effectiveness has been more intensely scrutinized than other health initiatives developed for adolescents, primarily because of the expectation that they could solve the myriad problems facing adolescents today. The trends found in this study indicate that, given the appropriate financial and community support, school-based clinics may be able to achieve the goals of improved health care and reduced risk-taking behavior among the students they serve. At the same time, the clinics will benefit greatly from opportunities to cooperate with other programs from diverse community organizations that also have been developed especially to meet the needs of adolescents. Reducing risk-taking behaviors and improving life options for adolescents are ambitious goals that require will, energy, and imagination. These goals can only be achieved if they are actively sought not only by the schools, but by a caring network that includes families and the larger community as well.

Prepared Statement of Faye Wattleton, President of Planned Parenthood of America, Inc., Washington, DC

I am Faye Wattleton, President of Planned Parenthood Federation of America (PPFA). I am appearing today on behalf of more than 30,000 volunteers and staff who operate our 172 affiliates in 46 states and the District of Columbia, the 300,000 individuals who contribute to our organizations, and above all, the more than 1.6 million adolescent women and men who are served by our clinics each year. I want to thank you, Chairwoman Schroeder, and the Select Committee on Children, Youth and Families for the opportunity to speak about risks to the health of American adolescents. I applaud efforts such as this and the recent Office of Technology Assessment's Adolescent Health report that encourage and facilitate discussion about how we can best serve the very real health needs of our youth.

The "Gag Rule":

I wish I could focus my testimony, and my organization's energy, on the ways that Title X family planning clinics can stem the tide of the health problems that plague American youth. Unfortunately, recent events threaten the ability of Title X-supported clinics to do so, and reopen adolescents to the host of perilous health problems that I will relate to you in this testimony.

The Supreme Court recently upheld the "gag rule" in the case *Rust v. Sullivan*. The "gag rule" is a set of Reagan-era regulations that would prohibit doctors and counselors in Title X-supported family planning clinics from giving pregnant women any information about abortion while requiring that all pregnant women be referred for prenatal care. The "gag rule" reverses a medical tradition of the commitment which the physician has to her/his patient to provide full information within the bounds of the law.

To allow the government to define the bounds of medical disclosure has profound implications for all, but will perhaps have the greatest impact on adolescents for a variety of reasons. Because adolescents lack the financial resources to obtain health care services through their own means, they are more dependent on government-funded health programs. Adolescents are also less able than adults to maneuver their way through the complexities of the health care delivery system to obtain their needed services.

As if the restriction on free speech in the context of discussing a young woman's legal pregnancy options were not bad enough, it is not the only likely effect the "gag rule" rule will have on health service provision to adolescents. Services providers who work with adolescents attest to the fact that adolescents' trust in their health care providers is a critical determinant of their continued use of health services. The "gag rule" will undermine the trust between the adolescent and the provider. Once the word hits the street that family planning counselors aren't telling the whole truth, adolescents may question not only the motivation of the provider but also the validity of all the information that is presented. Adolescents may view the clinic counselors as liars -- they won't differentiate that the counselor is not telling them the whole truth about pregnancy options and not withholding information about pregnancy, STD or HIV prevention. To the adolescents, the clinic counselors will be liars, period. This can only serve to weaken the motivation to use the clinic's services and increase the chance that the adolescent will be lost for all of the services provided by that clinic -- from HIV education to contraceptive services to nutrition counseling. Not only is there the risk that adolescents will be lost from the clinic's services, but since this may be one of the few, or only, contacts with the health care system, they may be lost from the entire spectrum of health care services until a serious illness necessitates contact. Therefore, the hopes of a few to direct women away from their legal option of abortion may, in turn, only serve to exacerbate a host of troubling and costly problems including STDs, HIV infection, adolescent pregnancy and parenting, and, through alienating them from contraceptive providers, increase the need for abortion.

Adolescents Are At-Risk:

The health and well-being of American adolescents are truly at-risk. Today's youth are facing health problems that are very adult in nature, yet they must maneuver their way through a health care system that is often unresponsive to their needs. The focus on their age has been used to deny adolescents needed services, rather than to call for adolescent-specific or age-appropriate programs to address their needs. American adolescents are doing the best that they can, but they need more from us to thrive. At the very least, we must provide them with all the information that they need in order to survive. Perhaps there are no better examples than those of the threats of adolescent pregnancy, sexually transmitted diseases and AIDS to illustrate how the "gag rule" will threaten our abilities to address the difficulties facing today's youth.

Adolescent Sexual Activity:

America must face the reality of adolescent sexual activity. According to research gathered by the Alan Guttmacher Institute, 50 percent of unmarried women and 60 percent of unmarried men aged 15-19 have had sexual intercourse. Teenagers are having sex for the first time at younger ages -- in 1979, 56 percent of unmarried men aged 17 living in metropolitan areas had had intercourse; in 1988, 72 percent. In 1982, 19 percent of unmarried women aged 17 had had intercourse; in 1988, 27 percent. Most of the increase in female sexual activity in the 1980s was among white teenagers and those in higher income families, narrowing previous racial, ethnic and economic differences. Six in 10 sexually active women aged 15-19 report having had two or more sexual partners.

Contraceptive Use:

Perhaps what distinguishes this generation of sexually active youth is that these young Americans are being less "adolescent" about their sexuality -- they are responding to the risks they face by increasing their use of protection. According to data from the National Survey of Family Growth, seventy-nine percent of sexually active teenage women use a contraceptive method - up from 71 percent in 1982. Fifty-seven percent of sexually active unmarried men aged 15-19 used a condom the last time they had intercourse, and among those aged 17-19 in metropolitan areas, condom use more than doubled between 1979 and 1988 -- from 21 percent to 58 percent. While these developments are encouraging, the unfortunate fact remains that adolescents are more likely than any other age group to be nonusers: One in five use no method. Adolescents need more contraceptive education, as they use contraceptives inconsistently and have the highest contraceptive failure rates of any age group. It is the nonuse and ineffective use of contraceptives -- problems born out of insufficient information and education -- that makes sexually active adolescents vulnerable to a number of health problems.

Teen Pregnancy:

It may be that the lack of an effective federal program that takes a realistic approach to adolescent sexuality and pregnancy prevention has allowed the problem of adolescent pregnancy and parenting to become so everpresent that it has nearly become one of the "facts of life" in America. I hope that the inadequate current program will not stifle creative pregnancy prevention and care programs such as H.R. 1398, the Mickey Leland Adolescent Pregnancy Prevention and Parenthood Act, which deserves serious consideration by this House of Congress. Each year, more than one million teenagers - one in 10 women aged 15-19 and one in five who are sexually active - become pregnant. That is approximately 2,740 young women getting pregnant every day - nearly two pregnancies every minute. By age 18, one in four (24 percent) teenagers will become pregnant at least once -- and more than four in 10 (44 percent) will do so by age 20. Eight in 10 teenage pregnancies are unintended -- nine in 10 among unmarried teenagers and about half among married teenagers. Nearly one in five teenagers who experience a premarital pregnancy become pregnant again within a year. Within two years more than 31 percent have a repeat pregnancy.

The number of teenage pregnancies and the teen pregnancy rate rose gradually during the 1970s but leveled off in the 1980s, in large part due to increased contraceptive use. Still, U.S. teens remain unchallenged at the top of the list with the highest pregnancy rates in the western world. American teens also have one of the highest rates of abortion -- four in 10 teenage pregnancies (excluding miscarriages) end in abortion. Twenty-six percent of all abortions in the United States each year are to women under the age of 20. Every year about four percent of women aged 15-19 have an abortion.

The "gag rule" will most certainly exact its cruel cost at the expense of the over one million American teenagers who become pregnant each year. At that point, these adolescents need care, support, honesty and trust more than any other point in their contact with the health care system. The effect of the counseling that these young women receive about their pregnancies will not just last for the duration of that counseling session, but will affect their future well-being. Adolescents go to a family planning clinic for medical advice, not the ideological viewpoint of a particular presidential administration.

Sexually Transmitted Diseases:

Not only does unprotected sexual intercourse place adolescents at-risk for pregnancy, but it also places them at-risk for sexually transmitted diseases (STDs). Approximately 2.5 million teens contract an STD annually. That is one in every six teens. Adolescents represent 20 percent of all STD cases. Youth who engage in sexual intercourse have a higher rate of STD infections than adults who engage in sexual intercourse. Since most STDs are asymptomatic and many youth do not even recognize the symptoms, this serves as a barrier to their seeking STD services, and can often lead to secondary complications. Certain types of STDs, such as chlamydia and human pampilloma virus, which can lead to infertility and cervical cancer respectively, can be treated before becoming disabling or deadly only if they are detected early. But the STD can only be detected if the adolescents have contact with health care providers. For some teens, clinics that receive Title X funds are the only source of STD testing and care; for others who are timid about discussing sexuality-related issues with their family's private physician, the clinic is their preferred provider. If the barriers of nonrecognition of symptoms and lack of access to appropriate providers are not sufficiently formidable, the mistrust of providers caused by the "gag rule" may be the final factor to drive teens away from STD services altogether.

AIDS:

Perhaps what makes me the saddest is knowing that 10 years ago I may have ended my list of risks that face adolescents who engage in unprotected sexual intercourse at this point. But now I must add perhaps the most disheartening entry -- AIDS. In the 10 years since the advent of AIDS in the American consciousness, the demographics of the epidemic continue to shift to claim a greater portion of Americans for at-risk categorization. American adolescents are not immune to AIDS. Due to the possible latency period of two to 10 years or more between HIV infection and the onset of symptoms, the number of reported adolescent AIDS cases is relatively low. This does not represent the severity of HIV infection in the adolescent population. In fact, the length of the latency period coupled with the fact that a large share of AIDS cases are persons in their twenties, makes it reasonable to assume that a large share of persons with AIDS contracted the virus while adolescents. As of December 31, 1990, 629 cases of AIDS among 13-19 year olds were reported to the Centers for Disease Control (CDC). The Department of Health and Human Services reports that out of the estimated 1 million Americans infected with HIV, 74,550 are young people between the ages of 13 and 24. The number of reported AIDS cases in adolescent women aged 13-19 increased 67 percent between December 1989 and December 1990 in the U.S. -- more than twice the increase among adolescent males of the same age for the same time period. In the past year, cases among adolescents attributed to heterosexual intercourse increased by 50 percent from 14 percent to 21 percent. According to the CDC, the rate of reported AIDS cases in the heterosexual transmission category among youth (14 percent) is almost triple that of adults (5 percent).

We know that the populations at greatest risk for HIV infection are difficult to reach. The importance of family planning clinics in AIDS prevention has been recognized in the Healthy People 2000 Objectives, the Ryan White CARE Act of 1990 and in pending legislation such as Congresswoman Morella's *Women and AIDS Outreach and Prevention Act* (H.R. 1072). Still, the "gag rule" will serve as a wedge of mistrust between these difficult to reach women and adolescents and their health care providers. If you thought you were at-risk or had a life-threatening illness, would you seek out the services of a provider who you know will not tell you the whole truth about the legal, medical options available to you? I would not, but I am fortunate enough to be able to afford the services of a private health care system. Others, many adolescents and women, do not have that choice.

Title X:

While I present to you the dangers that face American adolescents, I also can report that the Title X family planning program has been directly addressing these problems to the best of its ability. Title X of the Public Health Service Act is the core of our national family planning clinic network that provides subsidized basic preventive health services to approximately 1.6 million teenagers. In addition to providing contraceptive services (including natural family planning), Title X-supported clinics also offer health screening assessments and either simple treatments or referral for anemia, hypertension, cervical and breast cancer, STDs, kidney dysfunction and diabetes, among others. Clinics such as those financed through Title X often are the client's initial entry point into or, in some cases, the only point of contact with the health care system. The growing need for the contraceptive and basic reproductive health services provided by Title X has been met by shrinking federal commitment of funds. In fiscal year 1981, Title X was funded at $162 million, and after dipping to a low of $124 million in FY 1982, has been funded at approximately $140 - $144 million from FY 1985 to FY 1990.

But this is a snapshot of what these clinics were able to achieve while they were unencumbered by the mandated restrictions on medical information that will be brought about with the implementation of the "gag rule." I find it difficult to believe that with the "gag rule" in place, I will be able to provide such an encouraging scenario in the future.

It is more than troubling to see the potential impact of these regulations in a country that prides itself on its freedom of speech, bases its economic system on the idea of an informed consumer and celebrates its children as its hope for the future. It angers me to see ideological disputes override the health and well-being of our adolescents. I urge you all to support legislation to overturn the "gag rule." And I commend the members of this committee and you, Madam Chairperson, for providing the opportunity to discuss the challenges facing us in keeping our youth out of harm's way.

Thank you.

○

47-042 (224)

ISBN 0-16-037310-7

90000

9 780160 373107